PHYSIOLOGICAL PRINCIPLES IN MEDICINE

General Editors

Professor M. Hobsley
Department of Surgical Studies, The Middlesex Hospital, London

Professor K. B. Saunders
Department of Medicine, St George's Hospital and St George's Hospital
Medical School, London

Dr J. T. Fitzsimons
Physiological Laboratory, Cambridge

Respiratory Physiology

PHYSIOLOGICAL PRINCIPLES IN MEDICINE

Respiratory Physiology

Second edition

JOHN WIDDICOMBE

Professor of Physiology, St George's Hospital Medical School, London

ANDREW DAVIES

Senior Lecturer in Physiology, University Medical School, Edinburgh

Edward Arnold

A division of Hodder & Stoughton

LONDON   MELBOURNE   AUCKLAND

© 1991 John Widdicombe and Andrew Davies

First published in Great Britain 1983
Reprinted 1987
Second edition 1991

British Library Cataloguing in Publication Data

Widdicombe, John
   Respiratory physiology. – 2nd ed.
   I. Title II. Davies, Andrew
   612.2

   ISBN 0–340–55253–0

QP
121
· W54
1991

Whilst the advice and information in this book is believed to be true and accurate at the date of going to press, neither the author nor the publisher can accept any legal responsibility or liability for any errors or omissions that may be made.

Typeset in Linotron Caledonia by Rowland Phototypesetting Limited, Bury St Edmunds, Suffolk. Printed in Great Britain for Edward Arnold, a division of Hodder and Stoughton Limited, Mill Road, Dunton Green, Sevenoaks, Kent TW3 2YA by St Edmundsbury Press Limited, Bury St Edmunds, Suffolk and bound by Hartnolls Limited, Bodmin, Cornwall

CONTENTS

GENERAL PREFACE TO SERIES

Student textbooks of medicine seek to present the subject of human diseases and their treatment in a manner that is not only informative, but interesting and readily assimilable. It is important, in a field where knowledge advances rapidly, that principles are emphasized rather than details, so that what is contained in the book remains valid for as long as possible.

These considerations favour an approach which concentrates on each disease as a disturbance of normal structure and function. Rational therapy follows logically from a knowledge of the disturbance, and it is in this field where some of the most rapid advances in Medicine have occurred.

A disturbance of normal structure without any disturbance of function may not be important to the patient except for cosmetic or psychological reasons. Therefore, it is disturbances in function that should be stressed. Preclinical students should aim at a comprehensive understanding of physiological principles so that when they arrive on the wards they will be able to appreciate the significance of disordered function in disease. Clinical students must be presented with descriptions of disease which stress the disturbances in normal physiological functions that are responsible for the symptoms and signs which they find in their patients. All students must be made aware of the growing points in physiology which, even though not immediately applicable to the practice of Medicine, will almost certainly become so during the course of their professional lives.

In this Series, the major physiological systems are each covered by a pair of books, one preclinical and the other clinical, in which the authors have attempted to meet the requirements discussed above. A particular feature is the provision of numerous cross-references between the two members of a pair of books to facilitate the blending of a basic science and clinical expertise that is the goal of this Series. This coordination, which is initiated at the planning stage and continues throughout the writing of each pair of books, is achieved by frequent discussions between the preclinical and clinical authors concerned and between them and the editors of the Series.

MH
KBS
JTF

PREFACE TO THE FIRST EDITION

This book is intended to help students understand the basic aspects of respiratory physiology. For the medical student it should provide a preparation for the 2nd MB Examination or its equivalent, although the passages in smaller print give information in greater detail than required by most medical courses. The companion volume (Cameron and Bateman *Respiratory Disorders* 1983) will be of special value in illustrating the clinical relevance of basic physiology to medicine, and should prove particularly appropriate for students at medical schools where there is a degree of integration of the curriculum. For science students the text should give a basic understanding of respiratory physiology, but supplementary reading will be needed for those taking honours courses in respiration. The book will undoubtedly be used to prepare for that bane of student life – examinations. Readers may take solace in the fact that using this book provides them with an opportunity to examine the authors and possibly their own examiners. However, no two examiners have ever agreed on the exact scope and depth of an examination syllabus.

Many colleagues have assisted with the production of this book but we would especially like to thank Dr Paul Richardson and Professor Ian Cameron for reading and commenting on some of the chapters. We are also extremely grateful to Dr Rodger Pack for the micrographs, Dr Mary Davies for the learning objectives and Carolyn Hollins for her help with the manuscript.

Finally, we greatly appreciate the help of Mrs Rita Perry for typing and manipulating the many versions and revisions of the manuscript, and the publishing staff for their efficiency and patience in dealing with the unreliable authors.

London, 1983
JGW
ASD

PREFACE TO THE SECOND EDITION

Respiratory Physiology was described in the preface to the first edition as 'intended to help students'. This still is our primary aim. To this end we have enlisted the aid of a number of generations of student users of the book and asked them to indicate which parts of respiration they find particularly difficult and in which they would like further instruction. This has resulted in a number of changes in emphasis, usually involving slight increases in text. For example the neural and chemical aspects of control of breathing are now accorded a chapter each. The anatomy of the chest and the neuromuscular components of respiration which form the structural basis of any understanding of breathing have been included in greater detail, and the recent general interest in the upper airways in relation to obstructive sleep apnoea has been accommodated.

Respiratory physiology, like so many other branches of biomedical science, is developing at a tremendous rate. In the six years since the first edition enormous amounts of published works have appeared. We have gleaned what we hope is the best from these to provide a completely up-to-date selection of suggested readings for the reader who wishes to go further than our book can take him.

1991

John Widdicombe
Andrew Davies

1

LUNG STRUCTURE AND FUNCTION

The need for air by higher forms of life must have been obvious to the ancients. Anaximenes of Miletus (born *c.* 570 BC) stated that air, or 'pneuma' (literally 'breath', *Greek*), was essential to life. The function of air was open to speculation. Plato (428–345 BC) stated 'as the heart might easily be raised to too high a temperature by hurtful irritation, the genii placed the lungs in its neighbourhood, which adhere to it and fill the cavity of the thorax, in order that air vessels might moderate the great heat of that organ, and reduce the vessels to an exact obedience'.

Galen (AD 130–199) was probably the first person to have insight into the true nature of respiration, for he compares it to a lamp burning in a gourd: 'When an animal inspires it is, I think, similar to a perforated gourd, but when respiration is prevented at the appropriate place on the trachea, you may compare it to a gourd unperforated and everywhere closed'. With the benefit of modern gas-analysing equipment, Galen would have discovered that the respiration of animals is in fact very similar to the action of a burning lamp, consuming O_2 and giving off CO_2. It is the function of the respiratory system to facilitate this exchange of gases between the cells of the organism and its surroundings.

What is respiration?

The word respiration has come to have several applications. Physiologists use it as the equivalent of 'breathing' (spiro, *Latin*, 'I breathe'). Biochemists use it to refer to the oxygen-requiring chemical processes in tissues, cells and cell fragments. The vast subject of 'tissue respiration' will not be discussed here; rather, this book is concerned with breathing and the transport of gases to and from the lungs and tissues via the bloodstream. 'Respiration' integrates nervous control of breathing, the function of the lungs, the circulation of the blood and the metabolism of the tissues. It is therefore not surprising that the full study of respiration includes the traditional core subjects of basic medical science – anatomy, physiology, biochemistry, pharmacology and psychology. Even sociology could be incorporated since patterns of breathing, quite apart from speech and singing, can be a form of communication.

The basis of respiration

Microscopic organisms can rely on *diffusion* to carry O_2 to their cells and to remove CO_2. Most multicellular organisms are too large to allow diffusion alone to be effective – the distances gases would have to diffuse are too great to maintain life. Although in man the same passive force of diffusion alone supplies and removes these gases (there is no active chemical transport of O_2 and CO_2), it is aided by complicated respiratory and cardiovascular systems which accomplish what the surrounding pond water does for amoebae. These systems are susceptible to breakdowns, which are considered in the companion volume (Cameron and Bateman, 1983, see *Further reading* list). Here, however, we will concentrate on the normal functioning of a system which, with a lung volume of less than 10 litres, provides a respiratory surface of over 90 m² and can accommodate metabolic changes from rest to extreme exercise in a wide variety of environmental conditions.

The constant environment

To operate efficiently, the cells of our bodies must be provided with a stable environment, relatively independent of external changes and the activity of the whole organism. This is especially true of the cells in the central nervous system.

Neophytes in physiology often lay great stress on the role of the respiratory system is supplying O_2 to the tissues. This role is important, but of greater immediate urgency is the removal of CO_2, one of the products of oxidative metabolism. The importance the body places on eliminating this substance can be judged by re-breathing from a plastic bag for a few minutes. Most of the drive to breathe and the unpleasant sensation which forces you to stop this rather dangerous manoeuvre are due to hypercapnia (high concentrations of CO_2). Carbon dioxide is an 'acid' gas. It dissolves in body fluids to form carbonic acid which dissociates into bicarbonate and hydrogen ions.

$$CO_2 + H_2O \rightleftharpoons H_2CO_3 \rightleftharpoons HCO_3^- + H^+ \qquad\qquad 1.1$$

It is to keep its acidity (often measured as pH, which is $-\log_{10} [H^+]$ in $mol \cdot l^{-1}$) within tolerable limits that the body responds so strongly to any build-up of CO_2. Blood in normally maintained close to pH 7.40, in part by adjustments in respiration. Those who are overly impressed by the narrowness of the normal pH range (7.35–7.45) should remember that pH is on a $\log_{10}$ scale and so a change of one unit of pH means a tenfold change in $[H^+]$. If pH were to change by 10 per cent from 7.00 to 7.70, about the extreme possible range, $[H^+]$ would change 500 per cent from 0.0001 to 0.00002 mmol $\cdot l^{-1}$.

Circulation and respiration

The circulation of the blood is intimately related to respiration. It forms the transport link between the lungs and the tissues, the two sites of gas exchange. We shall see in Chapter 7 that the matching of blood flow and ventilation in the lungs is of prime importance to their efficient functioning, just as the balance of blood flow and metabolism in the tissues is crucial to their normal function.

The time courses of events in the respiratory and circulatory systems are rather different. At rest, your heart may beat sixty times per minute while you take only fifteen breaths. The gas in the lungs changes in composition during inspiration as fresh air is added to the reservoir of gas in the chest, and during expiration as gas exchange with the blood continues. Blood pulsing through the lungs absorbs these respiratory oscillations in gas tensions. In conditions such as exercise, not only will the size and timing of the cardiac and respiratory cycles be different, but both should match metabolism. For breathing, this matching is brought about by a control system in the brain which receives information from many sources, including sensors which monitor O_2 and CO_2 tensions in the blood and the extracellular fluid of the brain, and others that respond to mechanical changes in the lungs and chest wall. This information is used to determine a pattern of breathing which maintains appropriate blood O_2 and CO_2 tensions with the minimum expenditure of energy.

The lungs also have passive roles as an elastic liquid reservoir supplying the left side of the heart with blood, and as a filter with millions of capillaries which trap clots, detached cells, air bubbles and particles, thereby protecting the more vulnerable coronary and cerebral circulations from blockage.

Structure

Before we begin to discuss in detail the functioning of the respiratory system, we must know something about its structure. The respiratory system can be divided into extrathoracic and intrathoracic parts. The nose, mouth, pharynx, larynx and upper part of the trachea are extrathoracic and are therefore not subjected to the changes in pressure in the thorax brought about by contractions of the diaphragm and chest muscles in breathing. Inside the chest the lower trachea divides at the carina into the right and left main bronchi. These continue to divide by an irregular dichotomous (each airway dividing into two 'daughters' of different sizes) system into smaller and smaller tubes until the respiratory surface of the alveoli is reached. The dimensions of some of the tubes that make up this *tracheobronchial tree* are given in Table 1.1.

Table 1.1 Dimensions of some of the airways that make up the human tracheobronchial tree. Note the increase in cross-section and percentage total volume in the last few generations.

Generation	Name	Diameter (cm)	Total cross-section (cm²)	Cumulative volume (%)	Number
0	Trachea	1.80	2.5	1.7	1
10	Small bronchi	0.13	13.0	4.0	10^3
14	Bronchioles	0.08	45.0	7.0	10^4
18	Respiratory bronchioles	0.05	540.0	31.0	3×10^5
24	Alveoli	0.10	8×10^5	100.0	3×10^8

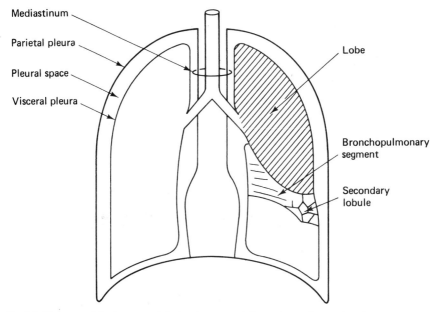

Fig. 1.1 Diagram of the lungs and their subunits and their relationship to the pleura.

It is interesting, and important, to note that while the airways are getting narrower they are getting far more numerous, so the total cross-sectional area is increasing enormously. Computer models show us that the angles between the airways and the dimensions of the airways are exactly right to cram the maximum alveolar surface area into the minimum volume. Each lung is anatomically divided into lobes made up of segments which are subdivided into lobules (Fig. 1.1).

The lungs lie on both sides of the mediastinum which contains the trachea, heart, major blood vessels, nerves and oesophagus. The lungs are covered by a thin layer of tissue called the *visceral pleura* and the mediastinum and chest wall are lined by *parietal pleura*. The pleurae are lubricated by a small amount of slimy solution and slip over each other during breathing.

The blood vessels of the pulmonary circulation follow the same pattern as the airways, dividing again and again until they are at the respiratory surface. Here the blood and air are in intimate contact, separated only by two very thin layers of cells (Fig. 1.2).

Nerves running with the blood vessels and bronchi control smooth muscle fibres in the walls of the airways and of blood vessels, and also the mucus-secreting glands. Nerves also conduct sensation and sensory reflex information in the opposite direction, from lungs to brain. The main nerves involved are the vagi (Xth cranial nerves) which travel from the brain through the base of the skull down the neck, through the chest to the abdomen (vagus means 'wanderer'). Sympathetic system nerves from the thoracic spinal cord also supply the lungs.

Lymphatic vessels drain the tissues of the bronchi and bronchioles, but not the alveoli where lymph capillaries might obstruct the passage of respiratory gases.

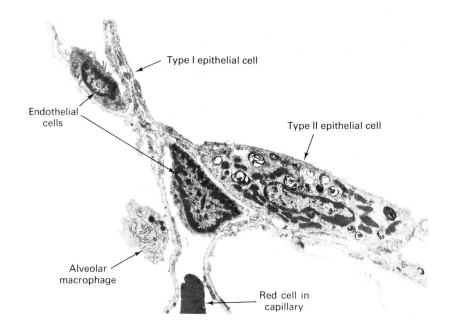

Fig. 1.2 Transmission electron microscopic picture of the alveolar wall. A Type II cell with osmiophilic inclusions is shown, and the epithelial extensions of Type I cells. The nuclei of two capillary endothelial cells are shown, with a red cell in one capillary. Within an alveolus, an extension of an alveolar macrophage is visible. (By courtesy of Dr R. Pack.)

Ultrastructure

At the *alveolar level*, there are capillary endothelial and alveolar epithelial cell layers (Fig. 1.2); the epithelium consists of flat Type I cells, and also Type II cells that secrete *surfactant*, a detergent-like substance that helps prevent collapse of the alveoli. The scanning electron microscope allows us to look into the alveoli (Fig. 1.3). Alveoli do not look like the regular balloons or bunches of grapes that are stylistically represented in some textbooks, but are pock-marked cavities with holes joining adjacent alveoli (pores of Kohn) and with macrophages wandering about ready to engorge and digest debris and foreign particles.

A scanning electron micrograph of the *bronchial* wall (Fig. 1.4) reveals a sheet mainly of ciliated cells which transport mucus up the airways to the larynx and pharynx, where it would be swallowed down or coughed up (Fig. 1.4 omits this layer of mucus). Interspersed between these ciliated cells are cells that secrete mucus. Deep to the epithelium is the submucosa, a spongy tissue containing blood vessels, lymphatics, nerve bundles, submucosal mucus-secreting glands and various other cells. Even deeper, we come to cartilage and smooth muscle. Figure 1.5 is a diagram of these tissues.

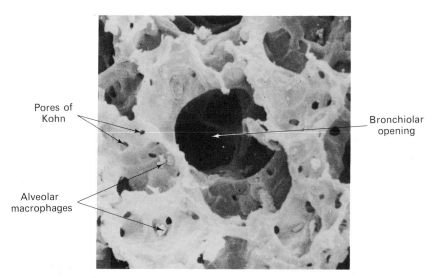

Pores of
Kohn

Bronchiolar
opening

Alveolar
macrophages

Fig. 1.3 Scanning electron microscopic picture of alveoli of a mouse. The lung has been cut across. In the centre, a large circular opening is the orifice of a terminal bronchiole, with alveoli visible in its depth. Other alveolar walls show macrophages and small holes (pores of Kohn) connecting alveoli. (By courtesy of Dr R. Pack.)

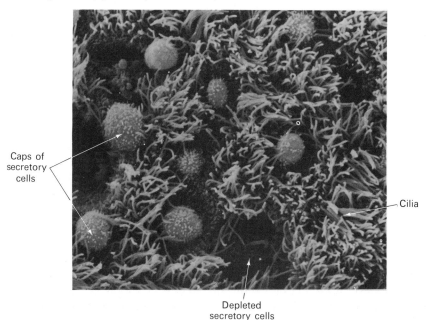

Caps of
secretory
cells

Cilia

Depleted
secretory cells

Fig. 1.4 Scanning electron microscopic picture of a bronchial wall. The cells are mainly ciliated, but secretory cells with prominent protruding caps are also visible. These may be mucus-secreting goblet cells. Their surfaces have microvilli rather than cilia. Denuded areas of the epithelium may result from cells have secreted their contents. In normal conditions, the mucociliary epithelium would have mucus on its surface, but this has been removed. (By courtesy of Dr R. Pack.)

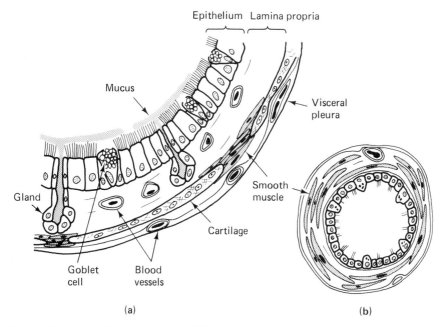

Fig. 1.5 Diagrams of (a) bronchial and (b) bronchiolar structure. The bronchus has a thicker epithelium and lamina propria, and also submucosal glands and cartilage. If, as shown, it is outside the lungs, it will have a layer of visceral pleura. The bronchiole has relatively far more smooth muscle.

How breathing is brought about

It is important to establish two facts before we go into detail of how breathing is brought about.

1. The lungs themselves have no muscles capable of causing breathing. The little muscle they possess controls the diameter of the airways (see Chapter 3).
2. Air only flows from a region of high pressure to one of low pressure. In inspiration, therefore, air has to be sucked into the lungs by reducing the pressure around them by increasing the size of the chest, and during expiration the pressure in the lungs is increased by a decrease in the size of the chest, compressing the gas in the lungs.

The diaphragm is a sheet of muscle that separates the thorax from the abdomen. It is attached by its outer margin to the lower edge of the rib cage and bulges up into the thorax. Each half of the diaphragm (left and right) is supplied by a separate phrenic nerve. These motor nerves arise from cervical segments 3, 4 and 5 of the spinal cord ('C3, 4 and 5 keep the diaphragm alive'). Activity in the phrenic nerves causes the diaphragm to flatten and descend in the chest like a plunger in a syringe, drawing air into the chest in what we know as inspiration. In quiet breathing, inspiration is the only active part of breathing; expiration is largely passive and is the result of the elastic recoil of the lungs pulling them and the diaphragm back to their resting positions.

The centre of the diaphragm moves about 1–2 cm during breathing at rest but may move up to 10 cm when breathing is very vigorous. These movements are responsible for about 75 per cent of the volume of breathing but are not essential for life. If the diaphragm is paralysed, other respiratory muscles can take over to a large degree. In quiet breathing, only some (and not always the same) muscle fibres in the diaphragm contract with each breath; this may explain the usual absence of fatigue in the diaphragm.

If the diaphragm can be likened to the plunger of a syringe, the ribs can be likened to its walls. The action of intercostal muscles on the ribs (mainly the 2nd to the 10th) can, however, alter the diameter of the chest and so actively draw air into and expel it from the lungs. This is largely because the ribs are set at an angle, sloping down from the horizontal but capable of being raised and lowered.

The intercostal muscles stretch between adjoining ribs, as their name suggests. There are two types, external and internal intercostals. The external intercostal muscles, innervated by segmental rather than the phrenic nerves, cause two types of movement during inspiration:

1. 'Pump handle' movements, in which the anterior end of each rib is elevated like the action of an old-fashioned farm pump (Fig. 1.6a);
2. 'Bucket handle' movements, in which the diameter of the chest increases, each rib on either side acting like the raising of the handle of a bucket laid on its side (Fig. 1.6b).

Both these types of action increase the diameter of the chest and thus draw air into the lungs. This inflow of air is due to a reduction of pressure in the chest. Not

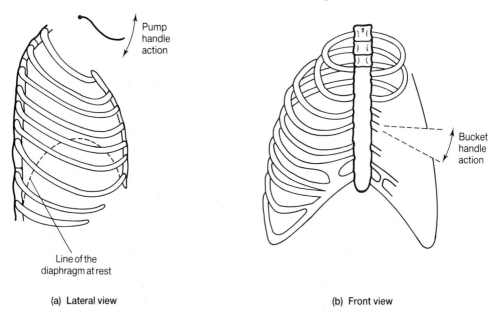

(a) Lateral view   (b) Front view

Fig. 1.6 Views of the rib cage showing how contraction of the intercostal muscles brings about changes in (a) the anterior-posterior and (b) the lateral diameter of the chest. For simplicity only nine–ten ribs are shown rather than the usual twelve.

only do the external intercostal muscles help to bring about this reduction in pressure but, by stiffening the chest wall during inspiration, they prevent the 'sucking in' of the chest (just as you can suck in your cheeks) that would take place if they did not contract. The action of the intercostal muscles accounts for about 25 per cent of maximum voluntary ventilation.

Although expiration is largely passive during quiet breathing (resulting from the elastic recoil of the chest and lungs returning them to their rest position), expiratory muscles contract actively during high rates of ventilation or if the airways are obstructed by disease. The abdominal muscles are the most important muscles of expiration. By squeezing the contents of the abdomen up against the diaphragm, they force it up into the chest, expelling air from the lungs. These abdominal muscles are especially active during a cough or sneeze, as will be apparent if you press your fingers into your abdomen and cough.

The internal intercostal muscles, like the external intercostals, occupy the spaces between the ribs and are innervated by segmental nerves. They pull the ribs down, reduce the diameter of the chest and so contribute to expiration. They, like the external intercostals, reinforce the spaces between the ribs and prevent the chest from bulging out during expiration.

The changes in size and shape of the chest brought about by the diaphragm and intercostal muscles (and several other similar accessory muscles omitted for brevity) are transmitted to the outer surface of the lungs. Because the lungs are so flexible, any change in pressure on their surface is rapidly transmitted to the air within the alveoli. This does not mean that the actual pressure between the layers of pleura that form the outermost layers of the lungs and the innermost lining layer of the chest is the same as the pressure in the alveoli (see Chapter 2).

Behaviour and breathing

Many of the functions of our bodies are carried out without conscious intervention. We need not be aware of our heart or kidneys, for example, for them to go on pumping and filtering the blood. The same applies to breathing, in that we are not usually conscious of its existence unless we deliberately think about it or unless we become breathless from exercise or disease. On the other hand, playing a trumpet, for example, requires modification of breathing and initially a conscious appreciation of what we are doing. A tyro-trumpeter will be taught to concentrate on his breathing; a professional will be unaware of it. Breathing is a function which carries on automatically when we do not wish to use the breathing apparatus for some conscious task; exercise is a similar example, in that we do not normally *think* how to make our muscles contract in running.

An illustration of the distinction between voluntary and automatic breathing is seen with some unfortunate patients who suffer from damage to the nervous system giving rise to a condition sometimes called Ondine's Curse, in which they can make conscious breathing movements but the automatic control of breathing no longer exists (see Chapter 9). Unless they are ventilated by a machine when asleep, they can collapse into a coma and die.

The respiratory muscles are used in a variety of non-respiratory ways to help other systems in the body. When you wish to move a heavy weight, breathing stops, the larynx closes and the chest is locked to form a rigid cage against which the muscles can act. The main respiratory muscles, diaphragm and abdominals, contract simultaneously to raise abdominal pressure in vomiting, defaecation and childbirth. Conversely, the respiratory muscles are switched off when we swallow food or drink, which might otherwise be inhaled. The respiratory system can help to cool you (mainly by evaporation of water) when you develop a fever. Changes in pattern of breathing can signal emotion, amicable or otherwise. Above all, we use the respiratory system to communicate by speech and vocalization.

Metabolic activity of the lungs

The lungs are more than a passive respiratory surface for the exchange of gases, powered by the activity of the muscles of the heart and thoracic wall. Because of their vast vascular bed, the lungs have a large surface area of capillary endothelial cells. It is mainly in these endothelial cells that a number of metabolic activities are found.

Naturally occurring blood-borne substances, such as 5-hydroxytryptamine, bradykinin, noradrenaline and prostaglandins of the E and F groups, are taken up and destroyed. Presumably this protects the rest of the body from possible adverse effects of these compounds, some of which would have been released from damaged tissues or from breakdown of platelets in blood clotting and passed into the systemic circulation. Other substances, such as adrenaline, prostaglandin A and vasopressin, pass through the lungs largely without changes in concentration, and thus reach the systemic circulation where their action is desirable.

Various exogenous drugs are either taken up by the lungs (imipramine, amphetamine) or are metabolized there (methadone).

Hormones and the lungs

Various hormones act on the lungs, and the lung releases hormones into the bloodstream.

1. The blood pressure-regulating hormone, angiotensin II, is formed in the lungs by the action of converting enzyme on angiotensin I; it is the same enzyme that is responsible for the destruction of bradykinin.

2. The lung releases prostacyclin (prostaglandin I_2) in response to damage to the lungs and in pulmonary embolism. Prostacyclin prevents platelet aggregation and thrombosis. This is sometimes called an endocrine action of the lungs since the prostacyclin is released from the lungs and is carried by the bloodstream to act elsewhere.

3. Several hormones act on the lungs. Steroids promote the maturation of some secretory cells in the fetus (see Chapter 2). Corticosterone and noradrenaline inhibit glucose utilization by the lungs, while insulin and adrenaline do the opposite. Insulin promotes protein synthesis in the lungs. The importance of these actions is uncertain.

Solids, liquids and gases

Respiratory physiology, more than many branches of biology, involves much physics. It should therefore be useful at this point to describe, at a very simple level, the relevant behaviour of three states of matter.

Molecules in solids attract each other strongly and are very tighly packed. Very few escape from the surface of the solid.

Molecules in liquids are more free to move and the most vigorous of them escape into the space above the liquid to form a gas which exerts a *vapour pressure*. Molecules in a liquid are, nevertheless, powerfully attracted to each other and, because molecules at the surface are attracted from one side only (the underlying liquid), they act like a skin and have a *liquid surface tension*. This is why small amounts of water form drops rather than spread out into a very thin layer. When a liquid surface is curved, as in a bubble, molecules in the skin are pulled towards the centre of the bubble. This is why bubbles have a positive pressure inside and tend to get smaller, and why they explode when pricked due to release of the internal pressure (Fig. 1.7).

Molecules in gases are free to move to all parts of the vessel containing them (molecules of the gases in room air do so at velocities of about $500 \text{ m} \cdot \text{s}^{-1}$). The attraction between molecules of a gas is relatively weak because they are far apart. The pressure exerted by a gas on the walls of its container depends on its temperature (which determines the velocity and energy of the molecules) and on the number of molecules present. Each member of a mixture of gases is responsible for part of the total pressure that the mixture produces. This *partial*

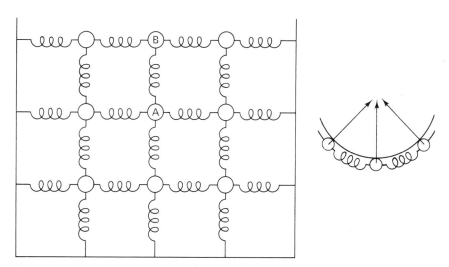

Fig. 1.7 Molecules in a liquid mutually attract each other. This attractive force is shown in the diagrams as springs. In the left-hand diagram the molecule at A is balanced by equal forces on all sides. A molecule at the surface (B) has no force from above, and the surface has a tension along its horizontal plane. If the surface is curved (right-hand diagram), the surface forces are resolved towards the centre of curvature which is why bubbles tend to get smaller and need a positive pressure to distend them.

pressure is proportional to the amount of that gas present. It is easy to see that in a cylinder containing only O_2 all the pressure is due to that gas. But in a cylinder containing 25 per cent O_2 in any other gas, only 25 per cent of the total pressure is due to O_2.

The vapour pressure of liquids, due to the escape of molecules into the gas phase, increases with temperature. In a mixture of gases, these gaseous molecules also exert a partial pressure. The only liquid that need concern us is water, which exerts a pressure in the gaseous phase of 6 kPa (47 mmHg) at body temperature. Air in the lungs has an absolute total pressure of about 100 kPa (760 mmHg), the same as amospheric pressure, so the pressure exerted by the remaining (non-water) gases is:

$$100 - 6 = 94 \text{ kPa (713 mmHg)}$$

This non-water partial pressure is made up of the 'dry' partial pressures of O_2, CO_2 and N_2. Nitrogen is conventionally regarded as including inert gases (Ar, Ne etc.) in this context.

Units

Medical science is at this moment in an unfortunate state of flux between metric and Standard International (SI) units (even Imperial Units refuse to lie down). In most places in this book we give both. The SI units are now standard in Europe, but are not uniformly or even usually accepted in the Americas. The only consolation we can offer is that the intellectual stimulation of having to grasp two or three systems of measurement may convince readers that physiology is a *quantitative* discipline and that we need to try to *measure* function. However,

---

Table 1.2 Some units of measurement in respiration.

Variable	Units SI	Metric	Conversion factor (metric to SI)
Force	newton (N)	$kg \cdot m \cdot s^{-2}$	1
Work	joule (J)	calorie	4.184
Power	watt (W)	watt	1
Pressure	kilopascal (kPa)	mmHg (or torr)	0.133
	$(kN \cdot m^{-2})$	cmH_2O	0.098
Surface tension	$N \cdot m^{-1}$	$dynes \cdot cm^{-1}$	0.010
Resistance	$kPa \cdot l^{-1} \cdot s$	$mmHg \cdot l^{-1} \cdot s$	0.133
		$cmH_2O \cdot l^{-1} \cdot s$	0.098
Compliance	$l \cdot kPa^{-1}$	$l \cdot cmH_2O^{-1}$	10
		$l \cdot mmHg^{-1}$	13.332

In this book, minutes (min) will sometimes be used instead of seconds (s). Litres (l) will be used instead of dm³, and 100 ml will sometimes be used in concentrations. For metric units of pressure, it is conventional to use cmH_2O for respiratory mechanical pressures, and mmHg (or torr) for gas and blood pressures. The mmHg can be converted to cmH_2O by multiplying by 1.36.

the units used are not important provided they are defined and the reader understands the different units and how to convert between them.

Table 1.2 gives some of the units of measurement and conversion factors used in respiratory physiology.

Symbols

The symbols used in respiratory physiology are easy to understand and are only used to shorten the text and to allow mathematical expression of relationships. Primary units such as volume (V), pressure (P) and flow ($\dot{V}$) are in given capital letters, as are those related to the gas phase (A – alveolar, B – barometric). Those related to the blood phase are in small letters (a – arterial, c – capillary). The primary unit is written first and then any qualifying symbol is given at a lower level. Table 1.3 gives most of the common symbols, together with a few examples of their combination.

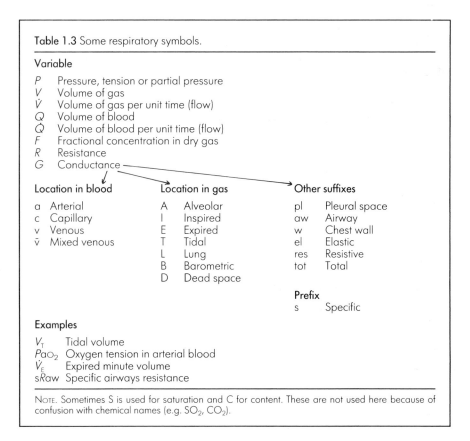

Table 1.3 Some respiratory symbols.

Variable

P	Pressure, tension or partial pressure
V	Volume of gas
$\dot{V}$	Volume of gas per unit time (flow)
Q	Volume of blood
$\dot{Q}$	Volume of blood per unit time (flow)
F	Fractional concentration in dry gas
R	Resistance
G	Conductance

Location in blood		Location in gas		Other suffixes	
a	Arterial	A	Alveolar	pl	Pleural space
c	Capillary	I	Inspired	aw	Airway
v	Venous	E	Expired	w	Chest wall
v̄	Mixed venous	T	Tidal	el	Elastic
		L	Lung	res	Resistive
		B	Barometric	tot	Total
		D	Dead space		

Prefix

s	Specific

Examples

V_T	Tidal volume
Pa_{O_2}	Oxygen tension in arterial blood
$\dot{V}_E$	Expired minute volume
sRaw	Specific airways resistance

NOTE. Sometimes S is used for saturation and C for content. These are not used here because of confusion with chemical names (e.g. SO_2, CO_2).

Laws

Physiologists, being modest and sceptical, dislike laws, but the study of physiology is nonetheless based on the acceptance of certain physical laws which illuminate the behaviour of the mechanical and chemical systems involved in respiratory physiology.

Gas laws

Boyle's Law states that the pressure (*P*) of a given mass of gas at constant temperature is inversely proportional to its volume (*V*):

   $P \propto 1/V$

Charles' Law states that the volume (*V*) of a given mass of gas at constant pressure varies directly with the absolute temperature (*T*):

   $V \propto T$

These two laws can be combined to give a general relationship between pressure, temperature and volume of a gas in different conditions.

The General Gas Equation, for a given mass of gas, is:

   $P_1 V_1 / T_1 = P_2 V_2 / T_2$

where 1 and 2 indicate the initial and final conditions being considered.

This equation can be applied, for example, to see what happens to lung gas volume when cold air is inspired and warmed by the body (at constant pressure), or what happens to lung gas volume when it is compressed by a forced expiration against a closed airway (Valsalva manoeuvre) at constant temperature.

Dalton's Law of Partial Pressure states that each gas in a mixture of gases exerts the same pressure as it would if it were present alone in the volume occupied by the mixture.

Thus, if a cylinder at 100 kPa pressure contains only O_2, all this pressure is due to O_2. If the cylinder contains 75 per cent O_2 and 25 per cent N_2, 75 kPa is due to O_2 and 25 kPa due to N_2, and these are often called the partial pressures of the gases.

Laws of diffusion

In a gas mixture, the lighter molecules will travel and diffuse faster.

Graham's Law of Diffusion states that the rates of diffusion (*D*) of two gases at the same temperature and pressure are inversely proportional to the square roots of their molecular weights (MW):

   $D_1 / D_2 = \sqrt{MW_2} / \sqrt{MW_1}$

where subscripts 1 and 2 refer to the two gases.

The molecular weights of the three main gases we breathe, O_2, N_2 and CO_2, are about 32, 28 and 44 Daltons respectively, so their rates of diffusion in a gas phase such as the alveoli of the lung are not very different.

Fick's Law of Diffusion states that the rate of diffusion of a substance through a membrane is proportional to the area (A) of the membrane, the solubility (S) of the substance in the membrane and the concentration gradient (ΔC), and inversely proportional to the thickness of the membrane (t) and the square root of the molecular weight:

rate of diffusion $= AS(\Delta C)/t \sqrt{MW}$

Respiratory gases diffuse faster across the alveolar wall or the tissue capillary walls if the area is large, the thickness small and the concentration (or pressure) gradient high. Carbon dioxide is 23 times more soluble than O_2 and has a larger molecular weight; it will diffuse twenty times more readily for the same pressure gradient.

Henry's Law gives the result of diffusion across a gas–liquid surface and states that at equilibrium the amount of gas dissolved in a given volume at a given temperature is proportional to the partial pressure of the gas in the gas phase. Gas taken up into chemical combination (see Chapter 6) is not involved in this balance, only that in free solution being concerned. If the pressure of a gas such as O_2 in the alveoli is doubled, the amount *in solution* in blood plasma will be doubled. The actual concentration of the dissolved gas is the solubility coefficient times the partial pressure of the gas in the gas phase, and the solution is conventionally said to have the same partial pressure of gas as that in the gas phase.

Gas flow laws

If flow is laminar, i.e. the fluid moves parallel to the walls of the conducting tube in an organized pattern as if in layers, the resistance to flow depends on the geometry of the tube and the nature of the fluid. The fluid may be gas or air in the respiratory system, or blood in the cardiovascular system.

Resistance $= 8\eta l/\pi r^4$

where η is viscosity of the fluid, r is the radius of the tube and l is its length.

Poiseuille's Law states that in such a system, flow ($\dot{V}$) equals the pressure difference (ΔP) between the ends of the tube divided by the resistance:

$\dot{V} = (\Delta P)\pi r^4/8\eta l$

This law applies in general to many flows in the body, but there are several qualifications that make its application imprecise. However, it is useful as an equation for measuring resistance of tubes such as the airways.

If flow is turbulent, Poiseuille's Law does not apply, as is discussed in Chapter 3.

Surface tension

Laplace's Law states that the pressure (P) inside a sphere of liquid of surface tension T is inversely proportional to the radius (r) of the sphere:

$P = 2T/r$

For a soap bubble, which has two surfaces, the relationship becomes $P = 4T/r$. For a cylinder, where the surface curves only in one dimension, the relationship for the single surface is $P = T/r$.

Measurement of gas volumes and concentrations

It follows from the gas laws described above that the same gas mixture may give different volumes depending on the pressure and temperature at which it is measured. There are two conventional ways of expressing volumes of gas mixtures and of the proportions of gases in them.

STPD means 'standard temperature and pressure dry', and refers to the volumes which would exist if all water vapour were removed and the gas were at 0°C (273° Kelvin) and 100 kPa (760 mmHg, 1 bar or atmosphere) pressure. It is used to standardize laboratory values for analysis of gas mixtures.

BTPS means 'body temperature and pressure saturated with water vapour' and applies, for example, to values of gas expired from the lungs.

If respiratory gas is collected in a bag at room temperature and analysed for O_2, N_2 and CO_2, these gases can either be expressed at STDP or at BTPS. The numerical values may be considerably different. In this book we will not make the distinction in the values given, since physiological principles are not affected by them, but in actual clinical or laboratory measurements it is essential to define the conditions you are applying when you give values for gas volumes, pressures and percentages.

Learning objectives

You should now be able to:

1. give a general account of how we breathe including the actions of respiratory muscles;
2. understand the role of respiration in maintaining the constant internal environment;
3. relate lung structures (macro- and microscopic) to function;
4. outline the non-respiratory functions of the lungs;
5. understand those aspects of the behaviour of liquids and gases which are important in respiration;
6. outline nine physical laws important in respiration;
7. identify the major symbols used in respiratory physiology.

2

PRESSURE AND VOLUME

Intrapleural pressure (P_{pl})

In relaxed expiration, with no contraction of the respiratory muscles, there is a negative (i.e. less than atmospheric) pressure in the intrapleural 'space'. This 'space' contains a few millilitres of fluid similar in composition to interstitial fluid. The negative pressure is due to the elastic contraction of the lungs (a recoil force) – if you take them out of the body they will collapse just as an inflated rubber balloon does when opened. At the end of a relaxed expiration, when airflow has stopped, this inward force of the lungs is exactly balanced by an outward force due to the elasticity of the chest wall. If the forces did not exactly balance, there would be movement in one or other direction, since both the lungs and chest wall are flexible. The presence of balancing elastic forces can be seen in surgery; if the chest is opened, the lungs collapse and the ribs spring outward (Fig. 2.1).

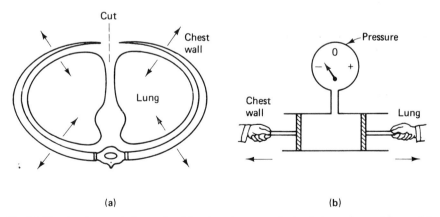

(a) (b)

Fig. 2.1 The development of negative intrapleural pressure is due to inwards recoil force of the lungs and outwards recoil force of the chest wall. (a) The direction of these forces and the movements of the lungs and chest wall that would result if the thorax were opened. (b) A model of how intrapleural pressure is generated.

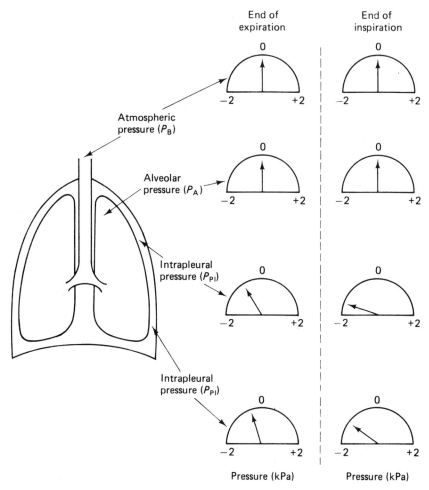

Fig. 2.2 The pressures in the atmosphere, alveoli and intrapleural space at the end of expiration and at the end of inspiration in a standing man. Note that only the intrapleural pressure is more negative at the end of inspiration, and that the intrapleural pressure is more negative at the apex compared with the base of the lungs. By convention, atmospheric pressure is given as zero, although at sea level it would be about 100 kPa (760 mmHg) absolute.

Pressure in the intrapleural space (P_{pl}) at the end of the expiratory pause of quiet breathing is about -0.5 kPa $(-5$ cmH$_2$O) relative to atmospheric pressure. It is important to understand that under most conditions (except cough, see p. 107) the intrapleural pressure is negative with respect to *both* the atmosphere *and* the gas within the alveoli (Fig. 2.2).

Although most animals have a small intrapleural space, it is not essential for healthy lung function. Elephants are said to lack one, and surgeons sometimes fix the lungs to the chest wall in patients with ruptured lungs.

If there were air in the intrapleural space, the pressure would be the same throughout. However, the presence of the thin film of fluid between the lungs and chest wall permits different pressures at different levels of the thorax due to gravity. The lungs are not made of rigid tissue and, if they were suspended in air by the trachea, they would behave rather like a concertina which, when similarly held, is more compressed at the bottom than at the top. Because of this property, the P_{pl} varies with the position in the intrapleural space where it is measured. For a standing man, at the end of expiration, the pressure relative to atmospheric would be about -0.8 kPa $(-8$ cmH$_2$O) at the top of the lungs and -0.2 kPa $(-2$ cmH$_2$O) at the bottom, a gradient of about 0.025 kPa.cm^{-1} $(0.25$ cmH$_2$O.cm$^{-1})$ – Fig. 2.2 – which is close to the specific gravity of air-filled lungs. Therefore, the bases of the lungs are collapsed relative to the apices when standing. If, instead, you stand on your head, the apices collapse and the bases distend. The pressure differences are smaller when lying down, although then the weight of the heart tends to compress the back of the lungs. Although P_{pl} varies with the height of the point at which it is measured in the chest, the pressure *changes* in a respiratory cycle imposed by the respiratory muscles are similar at all levels. These changes determine the ventilation at each level.

During inspiration when the diaphragm contracts, it enlarges the thoracic cavity and lowers P_{pl}; this in turn changes lung gas volume (V_L), by drawing air into the lungs via the open respiratory tract. If the muscle contractions are tonic, i.e. if they maintain the lungs at a fixed volume, the static relationship between V_L and P_{pl} can be determined. P_{pl} is seldom measured in healthy man but, because the walls of the oesophagus are very flexible, intra-oesophageal pressure gives a reasonable estimate of P_{pl}.

Lung volumes (V_L)

At the end of expiration, when the P_{pl} averages -0.5 kPa $(-5$ cmH$_2$O), the V_L is about 3 litres; this volume is the functional residual capacity (FRC). When someone breathes in as far as he or she can and holds the breath, P_{pl} decreases to -2 kPa $(-20$ cmH$_2$O) and V_L increases to 6 litres. Similarly, when the person breathes out as much as possible, P_{pl} will be -0.2 kPa $(-2$ cmH$_2$O) and (V_L) 1.5 litres; thus there is still air in the lungs, the residual volume (RV), even when no more air can be expelled. The limits to these static changes are the anatomy and strength of the respiratory muscles and the elastic properties of the chest wall and lungs. Chapter 3 will describe how larger pressures can be generated under dynamic conditions.

Changes in V_L can be easily measured with a spirometer, but oesophageal pressure measurements to estimate P_{pl} are not routine except in special circumstances. However, the respiratory muscles and the pressures they exert are usually normal in lung disease; therefore much important information about static lung properties can be obtained just by measuring changes in V_L. Figure 2.3 shows that in quiet breathing V_L changes by about 0.5 litres – the tidal volume (V_T). When a maximal breath is taken in, the increase in V_L (inspiratory reserve volume, IRV) is about 3.0 litres. A maximal expiration will then expel the IRV, the V_T and the expiratory reserve volume (ERV), the total being the vital capacity (VC), 4.5 litres in the example given. The RV in the lungs is about 1.5

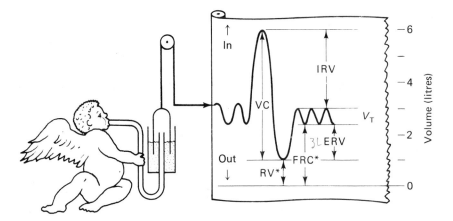

Fig. 2.3 Some volumes that can be measured with a spirometer, and two (FRC* and RV*) that cannot. The values are averages for an adult, and the abbreviations are explained in the text.

litres. If the lungs are taken out of the body and allowed to collapse, there will be still a little air left, the minimal air, 0.15 litres; these lungs will float if put in water. The lungs of a stillborn baby, who has not taken a breath of air, will not float; this has been used to diagnose stillbirth.

Figure 2.3 summarizes these abbreviations and their normal values for a healthy adult male. Whereas the pressures exerted vary little in health (and many respiratory diseases), both in man and in different mammals, the volumes vary with:

1. body size – all the volumes are larger in larger people;
2. age – the volumes are smaller in children, only partly because of body size, and in old age degenerative changes cause the VC to decrease and the RV to increase;
3. sex – all the volumes are slightly smaller in females, not merely due to the difference in body size;
4. muscular training – this increases all the lung volumes and allows greater maximal lung ventilation in exercise;
5. many diseases of the lungs and respiratory system (Cameron and Bateman, 1983). Normal values can be obtained from tables or equations for different heights, sexes and ages (Cotes, 1979).

V_T, VC, IRV and ERV can all be measured with a spirometer. RV and FRC (RV + ERV) cannot: they have to be measured by inhaling a known volume of a non-absorbable tracer gas (e.g. helium) and measuring its dilution when it mixes with the unknown volume of gas initially in the lungs; alternatively, the subject continuously breathes pure O_2 while all the expired air is collected in a bag and the total amount of washed-out N_2 is measured (since the alveolar gas started with a N_2 concentration of about 80 per cent, its initial volume can be calculated).

Static lung compliance (C$_L$)

Lung compliance (C_L) is a measure of the ease with which the lungs may be inflated. It can be found by inflating the lungs in a series of steps and by measuring the pressure required to hold the lungs at each volume. It must be emphasized that compliance is a *static* property of the lungs and, in contrast to resistance (see Chapter 3), it is measured when no air is moving into or out of the lungs. Although compliance can also be estimated under dynamic conditions, i.e. when the subject is breathing, all values and illustrations of compliance in this chapter were obtained under static conditions.

Compliance is expressed in units of litres.kPa^{-1} (or litres.cmH$_2$O^{-1}). It can be measured directly when the lungs are removed from the body or, in life, from the intrapleural or oesophageal pressures and spirometer volumes described above. Obviously, in life C_L below residual volume cannot be determined. Elastance (the reciprocal of compliance) is the measurement preferred by physicists, but is less frequently used in physiology or medicine.

Basis of lung compliance

Compliance is an expression of the elastic recoil force of the lungs tending to collapse them. This force is about equally due to two factors, the elastic fibres in the tissues themselves (see Chapter 1), and the collapsing force due to surface tension at the gas/liquid interface in the alveoli.

Surface tension in the lung

The alveoli have concave surfaces lined with liquid. In man, they are about 100 μm diameter at FRC. Such a liquid meniscus would tend to collapse the alveolus, due to the same forces that cause a liquid to rise in a vertical capillary tube. The physics of these surface forces is based on Laplace's Law, which states that the pressure exerted by a spherical liquid surface equals twice the surface tension divided by the radius $(P = 2T/r$ – see Chapter 1).

The surface tension depends on the natures of the gas and liquid. A bubble of 100 μm diameter, made of interstitial fluid and filled with air, would have an internal pressure of 3 kPa (30 cmH$_2$O). If you consider each alveolus to be such a bubble, vented to the atmosphere through the airways, you can see that the P_{pl} would have to be −3 kPa (−30 cmH$_2$O) just to hold the lungs open. Clearly, normal values of P_{pl} are much less. Either the alveoli have no liquid lining or the liquid lining is not interstitial fluid.

In 1929, van Neergaard described a now-classical experiment. He measured the compliance of excised lungs first containing air, and then with the air replaced by saline which would remove a gas/liquid interface (Fig. 2.4). The results led to three conclusions.

1. There is a gas/liquid interface responsible for about half the elastic recoil of the lungs, since replacement of air by saline doubles the C_L.

2. The liquid cannot be interstitial fluid because the pressures required to stretch the interface (difference between saline and air curves) are far too small.

3. With air in the lungs, the pressures needed for inflation are far greater than

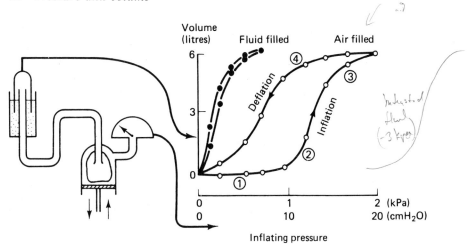

Fig. 2.4 Effect of a gas/liquid interface on the pressure required to inflate the lungs. As shown on the left, the lungs are inflated from complete collapse and then deflated, in a series of steps, by applying pressure to their container. Volume changes are measured with a spirometer. Thus pressure and volume are measured under static conditions.

For the air-filled lung, different pressures are required to hold the lung at a given volume during inflation and deflation, i.e. there is hysteresis. Note that the lungs do not significantly expand (phase 1) until a critical pressure of about 1 kPa (10 cmH$_2$O) is reached, and it then becomes easy to inflate the lungs (phase 2) until the tissue elasticity begins to resist (phase 3) at about 1.75 kPa (17.5 cmH$_2$O). During the early part of deflation (phase 4), the lungs tend to retain air while pressure falls considerably.

The left-hand curve is for fluid-filled lungs and shows that: (a) the inflation pressures required for any given volume are far smaller; and (b) there is no critical opening pressure and little hysteresis.

those during deflation. Thus, when pressure is plotted against volume for inflation and deflation, the plot is a loop – this phenomenon is termed hysteresis.

Surface lining of alveoli

The reason for the low surface tension in the alveoli is now known to be the secretion of surfactant, a phospholipid (dipalmitoyl phosphotidyl choline) with detergent-like properties, by the Type II cells of the alveolar wall (see Chapter 1). The surfactant spreads over the alveolar surface and into the alveolar ducts and bronchioles. It considerably reduces the surface tension of the interface. In its absence, and in some diseases (Cameron and Bateman, 1983), there is collapse of the lungs and pressures much greater than normal are needed for inflation.

The surface tension of surfactant can be measured by washing it out of the lungs, spreading it on the surface of a trough of saline, and measuring the force it exerts on a metal sheet dipping through the surface film. The film can be expanded or contracted by a movable barrier (Fig. 2.5). Although the surface tension of the surfactant film is always less than that of saline (or interstitial fluid), its actual value depends on its area and whether the surfactant film is static or is being expanded or contracted.

Type II cells of the lung first appear in the human fetus at about 20 weeks gestation, and surfactant secretion is established by 30 weeks. If born before that time, the infant may have surfactant deficiency which can cause respiratory distress. What controls surfactant secretion is unknown, but in the fetus its formation can be enhanced by corticosteroids, and we may expect to find humoral or nervous control mechanisms.

Opening and closing pressures of alveoli

If Laplace's Law is applied to a closed alveolus, it follows that high pressures are needed for initial expansion because the radius is small, and that these pressures decrease as the lungs expand. One might therefore expect C_L to increase as V_L increases. However, the pressure/volume curve for an air-filled lung is more

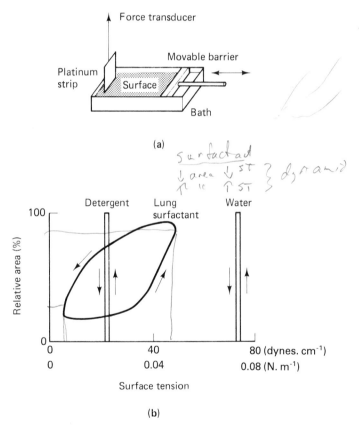

(a)

(b)

Fig. 2.5 (a) A device (Wilhelmi balance) for measuring the surface tension of a film of liquid with changing area. The barrier is moved backwards and forwards, thereby changing the area of the surface film, the tension of which is measured from the force acting on a vertical plate being pulled down by the meniscus of the film. (b) The surface tensions of water (high and constant), detergent (low and constant) and lung surfactant (low and area dependent) as measured in this way.

complicated because it results from the combination of tissue and surface tension effects (Fig. 2.4). It shows four phases.

1. High pressures are needed for opening collapsed alveoli.
2. At a critical opening pressure, a maintained inspiratory effort will cause inflation of large parts of the lungs.
3. After the critical opening pressure has inflated most of the lungs, increases in V_L require greater increases in inflation pressure.
4. On deflation, alveoli tend to remain open, and will empty at pressures lower than those previously needed to inflate them.

The presence of surfactant lessens the contribution of surface tension to the total compliance curve, and therefore decreases the pressure required to 'pop' open the alveoli at critical opening pressure.

The Laplace relationship tells us that if a large and small bubble are connected by a tube, the different pressures in the two would cause the smaller to empty into the larger. This does not happen between large and small alveoli for two reasons.

Firstly, the surface tension of the lining liquid of the lungs increases as the alveoli enlarge and decreases as they shrink, causing all the sizes of alveoli to exert about the same pressures. This hysteresis of the alveolar lining film is a characteristic of surfactant and can be demonstrated in the experiment illustrated in Fig. 2.5. Hysteresis contributes both to the critical opening pressure of collapsed alveoli on inflation and to the lessened tendency to collapse on deflation.

The second factor maintaining alveolar patency is mechanical interaction between adjacent alveoli or groups of alveoli. Collapsing alveoli pull on their neighbours, and the tissue elastic connections tend to limit collapse and stabilize alveolar patency.

Normal lung compliance

At FRC there are normally about 3.0 litres of air left in the lungs, which means that most of the alveoli do not collapse in expiration, i.e. we breathe at volumes represented by the middle and upper parts of the lung compliance curve. Figure 2.6 shows that the extreme hysteresis seen when the lungs are inflated from complete collapse (see Fig. 2.4) is absent in a tidal breath taken from FRC, and only moderate in a vital capacity manoeuvre. Even in health, at RV some alveoli collapse, but they are reinflated each time a deep breath is taken. This pattern is exaggerated in some lung diseases and in the neonatal condition (Cameron and Bateman, 1983, Chapters 3 and 4). The important point is that collapsed lung needs large distending pressures to inflate it.

Strictly, compliance is the slope of the curve (dV/dP) at any point. In practice, the mean slope of part of the curve, e.g. that in quiet breathing, is often taken. A healthy adult male has a compliance of about 2 litres.kPa^{-1} (0.2 litres.cmH_2O^{-1}), i.e. a slow breath of 1 litre would require a P_{pl} swing of 0.5 kPa (5 cmH_2O). Lung compliance depends on lung size (and therefore also on body size), so it is sometimes expressed as *specific lung compliance* (sC_L), which is compliance divided by lung volume at maximal inspiration.

Figure 2.6 shows also that the measured compliance and hysteresis of the lungs depend on the ranges over which they are measured. At large and small lung volumes (the ends of the sigmoid curve), the lungs are less compliant, and greater

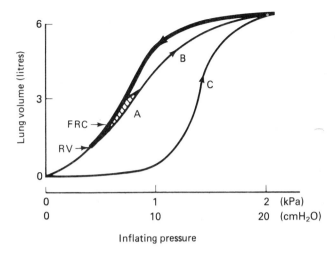

Fig. 2.6 A comparison of the pressure-volume relationships of the lungs during normal quiet breathing (A, shaded area), during a vital capacity manoeuvre (B, thick line), and when removed from the body (C as in Fig. 2.4). In quiet breathing, the lungs start from a partially inflated position (FRC) and little hysteresis is apparent. During the vital capacity manoeuvre (from RV) the hysteresis is greater, but still less than with initially collapsed lungs. The curves are drawn as if derived from static relationships, the dynamic factors described later in Chapter 3 being omitted.

pressure swings are needed for the same V_T. With a tidal breath from FRC the volume/pressure curve is much steeper, i.e. compliance is higher, than the average slope of the curve for a vital capacity (VC) breath. Also there is almost no hysteresis in a tidal breath, and only a little in a VC manoeuvre. This description may partly explain an apparent contradiction in the values presented in this chapter. We have stated: (1) that at FRC the P_{pl} is: -0.5 kPa (-5 cmH$_2$O) for a V_L of 3 litres, which gives an average C_L of 6 litres . kPa^{-1} (0.6 litres . cmH$_2$O^{-1}); and (2) that the normal adult C_L is about 2 litres . kPa^{-1} (0.2 litres . cmH$_2$O^{-1}). The latter is the average slope of the compliance curve over the whole VC range which gives a much lower compliance than that measured over a small tidal breath.

Chest wall compliance (C_W)

At the end of an expiration, the pressure in the alveoli is the same as that outside the chest, i.e. atmospheric, and the elastic recoil tending to collapse the lungs is exactly balanced by the elastic recoil tending to expand the chest. These elastic forces of the chest wall can be measured if we inflate an eviscerated thorax, in a similar way to the inflation of the excised lungs in Fig. 2.4. The elasticity of the chest initially helps inspiration. When the lungs have filled to about two thirds of vital capacity, the chest wall is at its rest position. Above that point, its elasticity produces an inwards recoil force resisting inspiration (Fig. 2.7). In a paralysed person it is possible to show this reversal and also to measure the chest wall compliance (C_W, the slope of the volume/pressure curve). In man, C_W turns out to be similar in size to that of the lungs, about 2 litres . kPa^{-1}

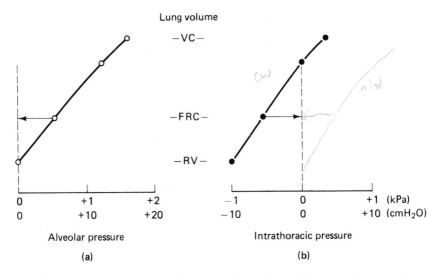

Fig. 2.7 The pressures required to inflate excised lungs (a) and the thorax from which they were taken (b) are compared at several corresponding 'lung volumes'. Only at functional residual capacity (FRC) is the pressure produced by the thorax exactly equal in value but opposite in sign to that produced by the lungs. The slopes of the two lines are approximately equal, indicating that the compliances of the lungs and thoracic wall are similar.

(0.2 litres . cmH_2O^{-1}). It must be stressed that the above discussion only applies to the *relaxed* chest wall, i.e. without muscle contraction superimposed.

It is anatomically more correct to speak of the thoracic wall than the chest wall, since the diaphragm and abdomen contribute to the total static forces. For someone lying down, the weight of the abdominal contents will press the diaphragm upwards, make the intrapleural pressure less negative and press air from the lungs. On standing up, the opposite will apply and FRC will increase. Unlike in the lungs, surface tension plays no part in C_w.

Total thoracic compliance (C_{tot})

Because the lungs fit inside the chest wall, like the rubber bladder in the leather cover of a football, the compliance of the *whole* system is determined by the compliances of the two components, which cannot be summed by simple addition. In such a system, to obtain total compliance (C_{tot}) we must use the formula:

$$\frac{1}{C_{tot}} = \frac{1}{C_L} + \frac{1}{C_w} \qquad\qquad 2.2$$

Because C_L and C_w are usually about equal in man, the compliance of the whole is only *half* that of each of its components. Thus, if normal adult lung and chest wall compliances are each 2 litres . kPa^{-1} (0.2 litres . cmH_2O^{-1}), the total thoracic compliance is 1 litre . kPa^{-1} (0.1 litres . cmH_2O^{-1}). It follows that artificial ventilation of a paralysed patient by positive pressure applied to the air in his trachea and lungs requires twice as great pressure changes as occur in his intrapleural pressure, or if his chest wall were opened in thoracic surgery.

Learning objectives

You should now be able to:

1. define the respiratory volumes that can be measured with a spirometer;
2. define those that cannot be measured only with a spirometer;
3. describe the factors that affect the size of these volumes;
4. define compliance and hysteresis;
5. understand why lung compliance depends on the size and gas volume of the lungs;
6. know why lung compliance is increased by filling the lungs with saline;
7. explain the significance of the special properties of the liquid lining in the lung;
8. understand the mathematical relationship between lung, chest wall and total thoracic compliances.

3

THE DYNAMICS OF LUNG VENTILATION

We have seen in the previous chapter that lungs removed from the body will collapse unless the elastic recoil of their tissue is balanced by positive pressure in their airways. This recoil pressure is *static* – it exists whether or not air is moving into or out of the lungs. To produce flow requires additional pressure, as air will only move through the airways from a region of higher to one of lower pressure. This additional pressure is related to the *dynamic* events of breathing, and it only exists when air and lungs are moving.

By far the largest part of dynamic pressure is used to overcome *airways resistance* to flow of gas. In addition, some dynamic pressure is needed to overcome the *viscous tissue resistance* of the lungs and chest wall. Lung tissue resistance to movement is only about one-fifth of total lung resistance (tissue plus airways). The *inertia* of the tissues and gases is only appreciable in large accelerations and decelerations of flow in acts such as coughing and sneezing, and the related pressures are very small compared with those producing airflow.

In a man with an intact chest, it is intrapleural pressure (P_{pl}), negative relative to atmospheric, that keeps the lungs inflated (not positive pressure within the lungs). During breathing movements, this negative intrapleural pressure can be considered to have two components, one due to the elastic recoil of the lungs and the other due to the fact that alveolar pressure must differ from mouth pressure if airflow is to take place. The concept of two components of intrapleural pressure may be easier to grasp if you visualize the lungs inside the chest as a balloon inside a large syringe, connected to the outside by a narrow airway (Fig. 3.1). It takes more force to draw air into the balloon (in inspiration) than to hold it stationary at any particular volume. Thus:

$$P_{tot} = P_{el} + P_{res} \qquad\qquad 3.1$$

where P_{tot} is total pressure, P_{el} is elastic recoil pressure and P_{res} is pressure to overcome resistance to airflow. When no movement is taking place:

$$P_{res} = 0, \text{ and } P_{tot} = P_{el}$$

During deflation (expiration), the recoil pressure 'assists' flow by squeezing the gas in the balloon, and P_{tot} becomes less negative than during distension. Note

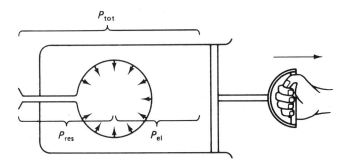

Fig. 3.1 While air is being drawn into the balloon the negative pressure inside the syringe (P_{tot}) is made up of two components. The first is the pressure required to hold the balloon inflated against its elastic recoil (P_{el}). The second is the pressure to produce flow along the airway (P_{res}). The pressure becomes less negative in two steps as we move the point of measurement from the inside of the syringe to the atmosphere via the balloon. The first pressure step is from inside the syringe to inside the balloon while air is being drawn into the balloon. The second pressure step is from inside the balloon to atmosphere.

that P_{el} is always negative relative to atmospheric, while P_{res} can be negative or positive depending on the direction of flow.

Types of airflow

Bulk flow of gas only takes place as a result of a difference in pressure. Flow may be *laminar*, when the molecules progress in an orderly streamlined fashion in the direction of flow, or *turbulent* when the molecular movement is chaotic.

In quiet breathing, most airflow in the lungs can be considered laminar, and the relationship between driving pressure and flow ($\dot{V}$) is defined by Poiseuille's Law (see page 15):

$$\dot{V} = (\Delta P)\pi r^4/8\eta l$$

where r is the radius of the tube of length l, in which a pressure ΔP is driving a gas of viscosity η. Flow obeying Poiseuille's Law has a velocity profile across the tube with maximal flow in the centre and zero flow at the edges. Flow tends to become turbulent if the gas velocity increases and if the tube becomes wider. Theory predicts that flow becomes turbulent when Reynolds' Number, which equals $2rv\sigma/\eta$, exceeds 2000 (v is gas velocity and σ is gas density). Under such conditions, flow varies with the square root of driving pressure and it is more difficult to propel the gas.

However, these flow laws only apply accurately with maintained steady flow in straight cylindrical tubes, and the airways of the respiratory system are not like that. Branching and irregularities in the shape of the airway walls, the churning action of the heart in the chest and the changes of flow associated with inspiration and expiration all dispose the system towards turbulence. Nevertheless, partly because of the difficulty of calculations involving turbulent and branching flow, the majority of physiological investigations assume that flow is laminar, which usually gives a reasonable approximation. Sounds such as wheezing in the chests of patients may suggest turbulence, but give no indication of its extent (Cameron and Bateman, 1983, Chapter 3).

Airways resistance

As pointed out earlier in this chapter, the relationship between inflating pressure and volume of the lungs is different if the measurement is made under static or dynamic conditions. This difference is the result of energy being required to produce flow in the airways and means that the inflation/deflation loop of inflating *pressure* plotted against lung *volume* is different under static and dynamic conditions (Fig. 3.2). The static relationship might be expected to be a single line, but in practice the static curve is a loop because of hysteresis due to the air/liquid interface (see Chapter 2, page 24). In addition, the pressure to produce airflow makes the dynamic loop even larger. The pressure to hold the lungs inflated at a static volume must only overcome elastic recoil, whereas the pressure under dynamic conditions must also produce airflow. By analogy with electrical resistance, we call the property of the airways which limits this flow *airways resistance*. Pressure is analogous to voltage and airflow to current. Applying the equivalent of Ohm's Law (electrical resistance = voltage/current) to the airways:

$$R_{aw} = P_{res}/\dot{V} \qquad\qquad 3.2$$

where R_{aw} is airways resistance and $\dot{V}$ is airflow produced by P_{res}. From Fig. 3.1 and equation 3.1, we see:

$$P_{res} = P_{tot} - P_{el}$$

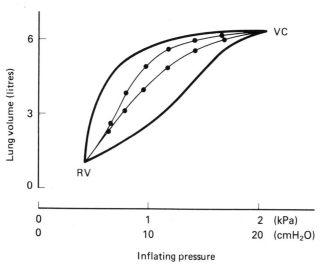

Fig. 3.2 The difference in pressure/volume relationships in lungs inflated and deflated firstly in a series of steps, i.e. measurements are made under static conditions with no air flowing (thin lines, as in Fig. 2.6B); and secondly under dynamic conditions with air flowing continuously into or out of the lung (thick lines). At any volume, the dynamic pressure is greater (more negative) than the static pressure during inflation, and smaller (more positive) during deflation.

Therefore:

$$R_{aw} = (P_{tot} - P_{el}) / \dot{V}   \qquad 3.3$$

This equation reinforces the important point that airways resistance can only be measured when flow is taking place. Equation 3.3 is another form of Poiseuille's Law, where $R_{aw} = 8l\eta/\pi r^4$. The units of resistance are kPa.litre^{-1}.s (cmH$_2$O.litre^{-1}.s). In a quietly breathing adult, a normal airways resistance would be about 0.2 kPa.litre^{-1}.s (2 cmH$_2$O.litre^{-1}.s). The resistance varies with flow rate, since higher flow velocities produce turbulence. A flow of 0.5 litre.s^{-1}, typical for quiet breathing, can be caused by a change in pressure in the alveoli of about ±0.1 kPa (± 1 cmH$_2$O). Note that this change is far smaller than the corresponding change in intrapleural pressure.

Resistance during breathing

There is normally negative pressure in the intrapleural space; this balances the elastic recoil pressure of the lungs when no airflow is taking place, as at the end of expiration. When inspiration begins, intrapleural pressure becomes more negative and this increase in negative pressure overcomes elastic recoil, causing the lungs to expand, producing negative alveolar pressure and thus airflow. It is important to remember that even with the respiratory muscles relaxed, intrapleural pressure is below atmospheric pressure and the changes in pressure which bring about breathing are superimposed on this.

The airways resistance of a human subject can be calculated if we measure changes in intrapleural pressure and the airflows they produce. Airflow at the mouth and intrapleural pressure are simultaneously recorded while the subject breathes normally. We know from Equation 3.1 (page 28) that

$$P_{tot} = P_{el} + P_{res}$$

and that

$$P_{el} = V/C_L$$

the static compliance relationship of the lungs (see Chapter 2), and since, from Equation 3.2:

$$P_{res} = R_{aw}.\dot{V}$$

therefore

$$P_{tot} = V/C_L + R_{aw}.\dot{V}   \qquad 3.4$$

If at each instant in the breathing cycle the pressure due to elastic recoil of the lungs (V/C_L) is subtracted from intrapleural pressure (see Figs. 3.2 and 3.3), we are left with the relationship between airflow $(\dot{V})$ and the pressure producing the flow (P_{res}) from which R_{aw} can be calculated; remember $P_{res} = R_{aw}.\dot{V}$ (Equation 3.2). Strictly speaking, this method measures airways resistance plus lung tissue resistance, but the latter is usually small.

The pressure due to the elastic recoil at any point in the breathing cycle can be calculated from the lung volume and compliance, which can be measured separately. In practice, all these steps can be carried out electronically (Fig. 3.3) and it is possible to measure airways resistance breath by breath. While

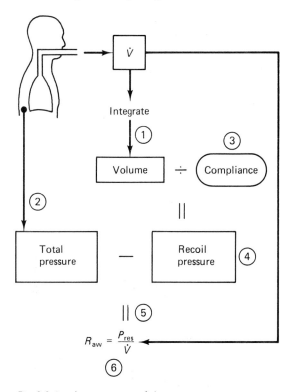

Fig. 3.3 An electronic way of determining airways resistance (R_{aw}). (1) Airflow ($\dot{V}$) is measured and integrated to give volume. (2) Total pressure (intrapleural) is measured with an oesophageal balloon. (3) Lung compliance is determined from the volume/pressure relationship at the end of inspiration (i.e. is 'static'). (4) Volume divided by compliance gives the recoil pressure of the lungs at any instant. (5) Total pressure minus recoil pressure gives flow-producing pressure (P_{res}). (6) $R_{aw} = R_{res}/\dot{V}$.

intrapleural pressure can be measured by introducing an air-filled needle into the intrapleural space, this is not very pleasant, and instead the pressure inside the oesophagus is usually substituted, using an air-filled balloon attached to a long thin tube. The oesophagus runs through the thorax, and its walls are so flexible that changes in intrapleural pressure are readily transmitted to the balloon. Figure 3.4 shows the changes that take place in a single breath.

Sites of airways resistance

About 50 per cent of the resistance to flow during breathing resides in the upper respiratory tract (nose, pharynx and larynx), and the change to mouth breathing causes a significant reduction in upper airways resistance. This effect is particularly important when flow rates are high and it is common experience that we change to mouth breathing while exercising, although the mechanism which triggers the change is far from clear.

About 80 per cent of the resistance of the lower airways (below the larynx)

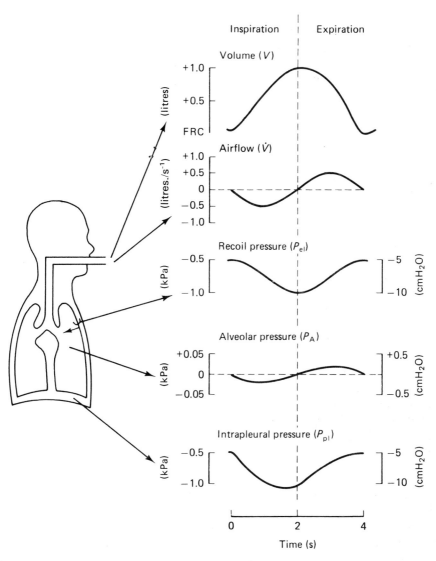

Fig. 3.4 Respiratory variables during a breathing cycle. Airflow ($\dot{V}$), volume change (V_L) and pleural pressure (P_{pl}) are measured simultaneously. Recoil pressure (P_{el}) is measured separately under static conditions; note that it is given a negative sign because it is measured relative to intrapleural pressure. Alveolar pressure (P_A) is calculated from ($\dot{V}$) and airways resistance. Theoretically, the curves for P_{el} and V_L are identical in shape, as are those for ($\dot{V}$) and P_A.

resides in the trachea and bronchi. This fact initially seems surprising when we remember that Poiseuille's Law (see page 15) tells us that the flow resistance of a tube is inversely proportional to the fourth power of its radius, and the trachea and main bronchi have the largest radii of the tracheobronchial tree. However, the reduction in radius of individual airways as they penetrate the lung is more than offset by the vast increase in their numbers; so the total cross-sectional area of the airways increases enormously (see Fig. 4.1). It is difficult to measure the resistance of the bronchioles and smaller airways, and they may be significantly damaged by disease before their abnormality can be detected by physiological tests. Although the trachea and larger bronchi are partially armoured against collapse by incomplete rings of cartilage, they can nevertheless alter their diameter greatly during conditions such as cough. It is the medium-size bronchi (2–4 mm diameter) which are the site of the most important physiological control of airways resistance. Their walls not only contain less supporting cartilage but also much smooth muscle which is innervated and can contract and reduce the airway radius. The diameter of these airways depends on active factors (e.g. bronchomotor muscle tone), on structural forces acting on the airways (e.g. radial traction), on transmural pressures across the airways, and on possible secretions inside. Each will now be considered in detail.

Bronchomotor muscle tone

The most important physiological control of bronchial diameter is by changes in tone of the smooth muscles in the airway wall. These muscles are mainly innervated by efferent fibres in the vagus nerves of the parasympathetic nervous system which cause contraction by releasing the mediator acetycholine. In healthy persons, vagal motor activity causes a resting tone in these muscles, which can be abolished by atropine (which blocks the action of acetylcholine) or by isoprenaline (which relaxes the smooth muscle). These drugs reduce airways resistance by about 30 per cent. The resting tone of bronchial smooth muscle can be influenced in a number of ways.

1. *Irritant, cough and C-fibre receptors* (see Chapter 9). Stimulation of these receptors in the lungs by inhalation of chemicals, particles or by disease produces a reflex with afferent and efferent pathways both in the vagus nerves. This reflex causes the smooth muscle of the airways to contract, reduces the diameter of the airways and so, in the case of inhaled stimuli, limits the penetration of the offending substance.

2. *Pulmonary stretch receptors* (see Chapter 9). These receptors in the lungs send impulses up the vagus nerves. Their activity reflexly reduces bronchomotor tone, so a deep breath may dilate the bronchi both by passive stretch of the airways and by reflex action.

3. *Carbon dioxide.* In overventilated parts of the lung, concentrations of CO_2 are low. These low concentrations act directly on the smooth muscle and constrict the bronchi, thus increasing local airways resistance and restoring the ventilation of that part of the lung towards normal. The response is direct and not a reflex action of CO_2.

4. *Mediator release.* In diseases such as allergic asthma, mediator substances that contract airway smooth muscle may be released. Many such substances have been described, including histamine, prostaglandins, leukotrienes ('slow-reacting substance of anaphylaxis') and kinins, but their relative import-ance is a matter of dispute (Cameron and Bateman, 1983, Chapter 3).

5. *Catecholamines.* Adrenaline and isoprenaline relax airways smooth

muscle, by an action on β_2-adrenoceptors on the smooth muscle membrane. Specific β_2-receptor stimulating drugs, such as salbutamol, are even more effective. Their use is the most common treatment for asthma (Cameron and Bateman, 1983, Chapter 3).

6. *Sympathetic nerves.* These produce the opposite effect to the parasympathetic (vagal) nerves, and cause bronchodilatation, probably by release of noradrenaline. Their importance is disputed, and the main nervous control of airways smooth muscle is by alteration in vagal tone.

7. *Other nerves.* Recently, other types of motor nerve supplying airways smooth muscle have been described, some of them inhibitory. Since their transmitters are not known, they are often called 'non-cholinergic, non-adrenergic nerves'. Their role and importance have not yet been established.

Radial traction by lung parenchyma

Airways within the lungs are surrounded by tissue (parenchyma) which pulls outward on them and helps to keep them open. This supporting action is called

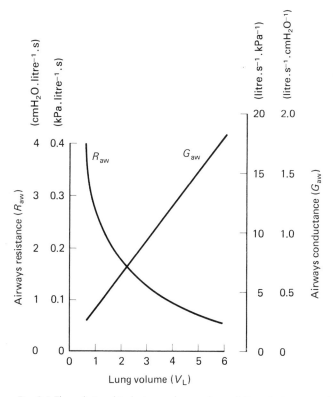

Fig. 3.5 The relationship between lung volume (V_L) and airways resistance (R_{aw}) and conductance (G_{aw}). At low lung volumes R_{aw} is high and G_{aw} is low. The relationship between G_{aw} and V_L is approximately linear and, since $R_{aw} = 1/G_{aw}$, that between R_{aw} and V_L is close to a hyperbola.

radial traction. As lung volume (V_L) increases, so does this effect. The influence of lung volume changes on airway diameter is particularly important at very low lung volumes since airways resistance (R_{aw}) may increase dramatically at these volumes, due partly to closure of some airways.

In practice, it can be shown that $R_{aw} \propto V_L^{-1}$ (Fig. 3.5). This relationship is important, because airways conductance (G_{aw}), the reciprocal of resistance, is directly proportional to lung volume and it is possible to standardize conductance measurements for differences in lung volume in various subjects and clinical conditions. Specific conductance ($sG_{aw} = G_{aw} . V_L$) is therefore frequently used clinically rather than airways resistance.

Diseases such as emphysema destroy lung parenchyma (Cameron and Bateman, 1983, Chapter 3). This destruction increases lung compliance, which might naïvely be considered an advantage. However, the loss of lung tissue reduces radial traction and allows airways collapse during expiration.

Transmural pressure

During *inspiration*, pressure in the pleural space is negative with respect to that in the alveoli and intrathoracic airways, and the airways are distended. During *expiration*, transmural pressure depends on the rate of expiration. If expiration is passive, intrapleural pressure remains negative and keeps the airways distended. If expiratory *efforts* are made, intrapleural pressure becomes positive with respect to the airway lumen and can cause dynamic airway collapse (Fig. 3.6).

Dynamic airway collapse results in *expiratory flow limitation*. The collapsed airway acts as a valve, and under such conditions increased expiratory efforts cause no further increase in flow. These conditions occur below functional residual capacity in health, but at higher lung volumes and with less extreme effort in the presence of obstructive lung disease where the airway wall is damaged or the supporting action of lung parenchyma has been destroyed. The collapsed segment of airway is unstable and vibrates. Its behaviour is highly complex. Wheezing during forced expirations probably results, in part, from vibrations of the compressed airways, as well as from turbulent airflow (Cameron and Bateman, 1983, Chapter 3).

The concept of an equal pressure point, where pressure inside and outside the airway is the same (Fig. 3.6), is often used to describe regions of airway collapse. At the equal pressure point in an airway, the patency of the lumen depends exclusively on the integrity of the airway wall and surrounding parenchyma. If these are compromised by disease, the airway is likely to collapse.

A number of tests of airways mechanics are based on measurements of volume and flow changes during forced expirations. These are described in the companion volume (Cameron and Bateman, 1983, Chapter 2).

Mucus secretion

Mucus or other material in the airways narrows their effective diameter. Mucus can be secreted from submucosal glands in the cartilaginous airways in response to reflexes involving vagal motor nerves with acetylcholine as the main transmit-

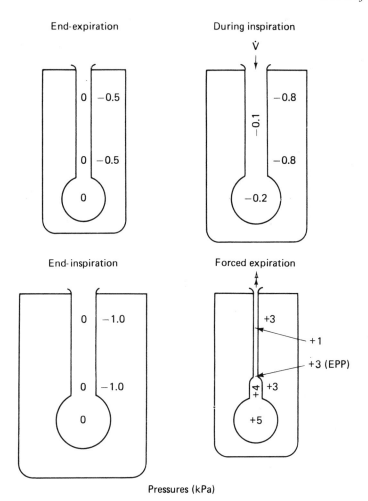

End-expiration

During inspiration

End-inspiration

Forced expiration

Pressures (kPa)

Fig. 3.6 Transmural airways pressures at different times in the respiratory cycle. A single alveolus and airway are shown, and the pressures in all the alveoli surrounding the airway are assumed to be equal. Note that only during forced expiration does an equal pressure point (EPP) exist and there is a collapsing pressure on the airway downstream from this point.

ter. Most people eating hot curry have a secretion of mucus by these reflexes. Mucus also comes from goblet cells in the epithelium of the airways, which can be made to secrete by local chemical stimulation. Cigarette smoke causes secretion by both actions.

Work of breathing

Mechanical work

In physical terms, work = force × distance moved. It follows that no mechanical work is done without movement. In a three-dimensional system,

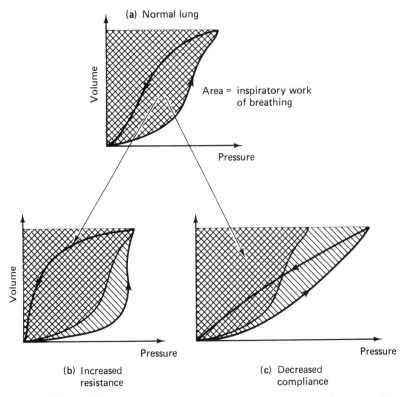

Fig. 3.7 Effect of (b) increasing airways resistance or (c) decreasing lung compliance on the inspiratory work of breathing. Inspiratory work of breathing is shaded area above each pressure/volume curve. In this diagram, the normal curve (a) is superimposed on those representing increased resistance and decreased compliance. Note that both increased resistance and decreased compliance increase the inspiratory work of breathing.

work = pressure × change in volume, and this equation is directly applicable to the respiratory system. In a diagram relating lung volume change to intrapleural pressure change (Fig. 3.7), work is proportional to the area of the graph. In quiet breathing, expiration is passive and the work expended is from elastic energy stored in the lungs and chest wall during inspiration. Energy for inspiration is provided by the active contraction of the diaphragm and other inspiratory muscles. Figure 3.7 shows how this inspiratory work would increase if there were either an increase in airways resistance or a decrease in lung compliance.

Some patterns of breathing are uneconomical in the sense that excessive mechanical work has to be performed to bring about a given alveolar ventilation. Thus, a minute ventilation of 8 litres . min^{-1} could be achieved by breaths of 2 litres every 15 s, 1 litre every 7.5 s, 0.5 litres every 3.75 s etc. (Alveolar ventilations would be slightly different due to wasted ventilation of dead space). Breathing which is very slow and deep requires more mechanical work because more work must be done to expand the lungs against elastic forces, while very rapid shallow breathing is also wasteful because more work must be done to overcome airways resistance (Fig. 3.8). It has been proposed that stretch receptors in the lungs sense the mechanical conditions there (Chapter 9) and adjust the breathing pattern to economize work.

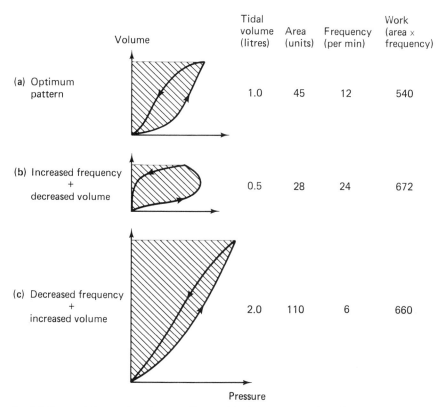

		Tidal volume (litres)	Area (units)	Frequency (per min)	Work (area × frequency)
(a)	Optimum pattern	1.0	45	12	540
(b)	Increased frequency + decreased volume	0.5	28	24	672
(c)	Decreased frequency + increased volume	2.0	110	6	660

Fig. 3.8 The work done in breathing is influenced by the pattern used. Inefficient patterns (b) and (c) of achieving the same minute ventilation are compared with a more economical pattern (a). The shaded areas above the curves represent the inspiratory work of a single breath and must be multiplied by breathing frequency to calculate work per minute.

Metabolic work

At rest, the activity of the respiratory muscles accounts for only about 5 per cent of the energy used in metabolism. By comparing the metabolic activity of the respiratory muscles with the mechanical work they perform on the lungs and chest, one can calculate their percentage efficiency, as for other muscles.

$$\text{Efficiency} = \frac{\text{mechanical work}}{\text{energy consumption}} \times 100$$

The efficiency in quiet breathing is low, less than 10 per cent.

In lung or chest disease, the work of breathing can increase very greatly, and a point can be reached where the increased oxygen uptake due to increased ventilation is all used up by the respiratory muscles; this must make hypoxia more severe and impose a limit on ventilation and total metabolic rate.

Learning objectives

You should now be able to:

1. define airways resistance;
2. know the importance of the radius (r) of a tube in determining its resistance;
3. describe the distribution of resistance in the respiratory tract;
4. know why resistance is a dynamic property;
5. describe the mechanical and physiological factors that determine airways resistance;
6. discuss the factors that influence bronchial smooth muscle tone;
7. explain airways collapse in forced expiration, and equal pressure points;
8. define work of breathing;
9. relate pattern of breathing to the work involved.

4

LUNG VENTILATION

In normal quiet breathing we take about twelve breaths a minute (respiratory frequency), each of about 0.5 litres (tidal volume); this makes up a minute ventilation of 6 litres . min^{-1}. Not all this ventilation contributes to the exchange of CO_2 and O_2, since some of it goes to 'dead space', containing gas which, unlike that in functional alveoli, is not in intimate contact with the blood. Air in the alveoli rapidly loses O_2 to, and gains CO_2 from, the blood in pulmonary capillaries which virtually surround the air spaces and together with the alveolar epithelium make up the respiratory surface.

The path of gas to the respiratory surface

Nose and mouth

During quiet breathing the healthy person breathes through the nose. The disadvantage of its high resistance, which is over twice that of the mouth and nearly half the resistance of the total respiratory tract, is offset by its efficient air conditioning and filtering (see Chapter 10). Many species, such as the rabbit, breathe only through the nose and can chew and swallow food at the same time as they breathe. These animals have lateral food channels in the larynx that functionally bypass the breathing channel connecting the trachea, larynx and nose. Some aquatic mammals, such as dolphins, have complete anatomical separation of food and gas channels, with a breathing orifice at the back of the head. Newborn babies have difficulty in breathing through the mouth and may become distressed or even die if the nose is blocked.

Pharynx

The pharynx extends from the end of the hard palate in the nasal cavity down to the larynx. It can therefore be divided into the nasopharynx (behind the soft palate), the oropharynx (behind the tongue) and the laryngopharynx (behind the epiglottis, see Fig. 4.1). The pharynx is of particular interest as it is the only part of the respiratory tract which is permanently shared with the digestive tract. In

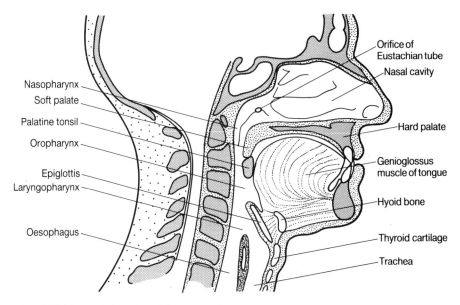

Fig. 4.1 Mid saggital section of the upper airways.

humans, the mouth is used for respiration in some circumstances, as in exercise or when the nose is blocked. The anatomical peculiarity of the pharynx as a region surrounded by soft tissue and not supported by bone and cartilage makes it a region very susceptible to obstruction: by foreign bodies, by swelling of the tissues due to infection and particularly during sleep due to relaxation of the pharyngeal and tongue muscles which hold the airway open; and this obstruction can result in snoring or the more sinister obstructive sleep apnoea (see Chapter 10).

Larynx

The larynx acts as a valve to prevent food and liquids entering the trachea during swallowing. The nervous control of swallowing is closely linked with that of breathing. During swallowing in man, breathing is interrupted, and every swallow is followed by an expiration. The larynx is a major and variable site of airflow resistance and, like the nose, a source of powerful respiratory reflexes.

Tracheobronchial tree

The tracheobronchial tree consists of an *irregular, dichotomously branching* series of tubes, making up about twenty-four generations in man. These are listed in Table 1.1 (Chapter 1). A plot of total cross-sectional area against distance into the bronchial tree is shown in Fig. 4.2. The peculiar shape of this plot results from the airways of the lungs increasing in number, due to branching, more rapidly than they decrease in diameter. Two important conclusions can be drawn.

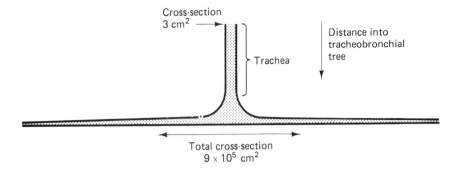

Fig. 4.2 The way total cross-sectional area of the airways increases with penetration deeper into the tracheobronchial tree. The final horizontal line represents the alveolar gas exchange surface, but is not to scale because it should be 300 000 times larger than the cross-sectional area of the trachea.

1. Deep in the lungs the total cross-sectional area increases enormously.
2. Most volume resides in the last few generations, since volume is proportional to cross-sectional area. This increase in volume occurs in spite of the small airways being shorter in length.

The functional consequence of these facts is that inspired gas moves very rapidly by bulk flow in the larger airways but far more slowly in the smaller airways until, in the alveoli, there is molecular diffusion to the respiratory surface. The implications of this pattern in relation to airways resistance are discussed in Chapter 3.

Dead space

Since essentially all gas exchange takes place at the alveolar surface, the tubes connecting this to the atmosphere can be considered *anatomical dead space*. Ventilating this region is an inescapable waste of effort as far as gas exchange is concerned. The concept of anatomical dead space depends on understanding the sequential filling and emptying of the lungs.

At the end of inspiration the alveoli have had their contents diluted by the room air, while only the latter remains in the dead space (Fig. 4.3c). When the lungs are now emptied, the rule 'last in, first out' holds and the dead space containing unmodified room air is exhaled first. At the end of expiration the anatomical dead space is filled with alveolar air, and this partly used air is inhaled first in the next inspiration (Fig. 4.3a and b). If some regions of the lungs are ventilated earlier in inspiration than others, they will receive more of this dead space gas; the regions receiving air later in inspiration will receive more fresh air. In other words, the timing of inflation of different parts of the lungs will affect the composition of gas they receive.

The strict definition of anatomical dead space is 'the volume of an inspired breath which has not mixed with the gas in the alveoli'. It is anatomical because it measures the anatomical volume of the conducting airways leading up to the alveoli. It can be

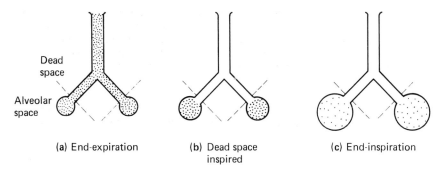

(a) End-expiration   (b) Dead space inspired   (c) End-inspiration

Fig. 4.3 The effect of dead space during inspiration. (a) At the end of expiration the anatomical dead space contains gas whose composition is essentially the same as the last gas expired through the lips, i.e. alveolar gas. (b) At the end of an inspiration of the same volume as dead space, the airways contain room air and the alveolar composition is essentially unchanged. (c) At the end of a deeper inspiration the dead space contains air whose composition is similar to room air, and the alveolar gas has been diluted by room air. A still larger inspiration would dilute the alveolar gas more, but would not change the composition of dead space air which remains like room air.

measured from the volume of expired gas leaving the mouth and nose before the 'front' of alveolar gas containing CO_2 arrives at the lips (fig. 4.4).

So far we have dealt with dead space resulting from the structures required to transport air from the nose or mouth through the trachea to several million alveoli. In the alveoli, air rapidly equilibrates with capillary blood. If some alveoli lack a blood supply, their ventilation becomes futile since no gas exchange is possible. These regions plus anatomical dead space make up the *physiological dead space*. With a healthy subject, anatomical and physiological dead spaces are very nearly equal, but in lung diseases physiological dead space can greatly exceed anatomical dead space because some alveoli are not adequately perfused and part of their ventilation is 'wasted'.

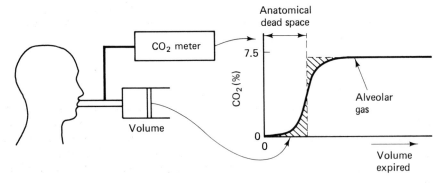

Fig. 4.4 The way in which anatomical dead space can be estimated when CO_2 concentration at the mouth is measured during a single expired breath. The volume expired at the time when the CO_2 concentration increases is obtained from a separate spirometer record. The flat portion of the graph, representing alveolar gas, is sometimes called the alveolar plateau. The vertical interrupted line is drawn so that the two shaded areas are equal.

The strict definition of physiological dead space is 'the volume of an inspired breath which has not taken part in gas exchange', and it is physiological because it assesses one of the functions of the lungs – gas exchange. It can be estimated using the Bohr equation, which is derived from the fact that the volume of gas expired (V_E) equals the volume from the dead space (V_D) plus the volume from the alveoli (V_A),

$$V_E = V_D + V_A \qquad\qquad 4.1$$

The total amount of a gas in an expired breath is the volume of that breath times its fractional concentration $(V_E . F_E)$. This total is made up of the amount from the dead space $(V_D . F_D)$ plus the amount from the alveoli $(V_A . F_A)$.

$$V_E . F_E = V_D . F_D + V_A . F_A \qquad\qquad 4.2$$

If there is none of the gas (e.g. CO_2) in the dead space, $F_D = 0$ and the equation becomes

$$V_E . F_E = V_A . F_A \qquad\qquad 4.3$$

or $\quad V_A = \dfrac{V_E . F_E}{F_A} \qquad\qquad 4.4$

Since $V_A = V_E - V_D$ (from Equation 4.1), then:

$$V_E - V_D = \frac{V_E . F_E}{F_A} \qquad\qquad 4.5$$

or $\quad V_D = V_E - \dfrac{V_E . F_E}{F_A} \qquad\qquad 4.6$

or $\quad V_D = V_E \left(1 - \dfrac{F_E}{F_A} \right) \qquad\qquad 4.7$

This is a simplified Bohr equation for CO_2.

So, by knowing the volume of air expired, the concentration of CO_2 in it and the concentration of CO_2 in alveolar air, we can calculate dead space. A sample of alveolar air is most easily obtained by getting the subject to expire down a long narrow tube; the gas in the tube at the end of expiration is alveolar air (essentially as for Fig. 4.4). The Bohr equation can also be applied to O_2 values, or for any gas involved in alveolar gas exchange. A major problem is that the use of end-expired gas tensions to indicate average alveolar values is not very accurate and, for CO_2, arterial P_{CO_2} may be a better index of mixed alveolar P_{CO_2}.

Size of dead space

Both anatomical and physiological dead spaces are about 150 ml in a normal adult. They vary with total lung volume in an approximately linear fashion. Thus, as lung volume increases from a normal FRC of 3 litres to 6 litres (near vital capacity), dead space volume will double. It follows that dead space volume varies with body size, age, sex and physical training, all of which influence lung volume.

Surprisingly, physiological dead space varies also with pattern of breathing. Breath-holding reduces measured dead space by increasing the time available for diffusion in the bronchioles and for the mixing action of the movement of the heart. Even if you breathe out immediately after inspiration, the last gas expelled has been subjected to a longer 'breath-holding' compared with that expelled first.

In theory, a tidal volume of 150 ml should not ventilate the lungs at all but, if breathing is very rapid, axial streaming of air partially ventilates the alveoli and allows gas exchange, and we have the paradox that physiological dead space is smaller than the volume of the conducting airways; it is clear that dead space measurements must be interpreted with caution.

Alveolar ventilation

Only that part of minute ventilation that reaches the alveoli and takes part in exchange of oxygen and carbon dioxide is useful in terms of respiration. From equation 4.1 we can obtain:

$$fV_E = f(V_D + V_A) \qquad\qquad 4.8$$

where f is frequency of breathing, or

$$\dot{V}_A = \dot{V}_E - \dot{V}_D \qquad\qquad 4.9$$

where $\dot{V}_A$, $\dot{V}_E$ and $\dot{V}_D$ are alveolar, minute and dead space ventilations respectively.

In an average healthy adult at rest, V_A is about 0.35 litres ($V_T = 0.5$ and $V_D = 0.15$ litres), and thus $\dot{V}_A$ is 4.2 litre.min^{-1}, for a breathing frequency of 12/min. Room air contains 21 per cent O_2, and alveolar gas about 14 per cent O_2, so the O_2 uptake is $4.2 \times (21 - 14)/100$ litre.min^{-1} or 294 ml.min^{-1}. For CO_2, corresponding values are 0 per cent for room air and 5.5 per cent for alveolar gas, giving CO_2 output of $4.2 \times (5.5 - 0)/100 = 231$ ml.min^{-1}. These are representative values given as an illustration.

The ratio of CO_2 output divided by O_2 uptake is called the respiratory exchange ratio, or respiratory quotient, and is often symbolized as R. At rest it can range from 1.0 to 0.7, depending on the food being metabolized: carbohydrate gives an R of 1.0, fat of 0.7 and protein about 0.8. For the figures given above, $R = 231/294 = 0.79$. We will see in Chapter 10 how alveolar gas exchange can vary in exercise.

Distribution of inspired gas

You may have noted from Fig. 4.4 that CO_2 concentration does not rise as a sudden step to its alveolar value. This effect is due to a combination of several factors.

Fluid flow in a tube is either (a) laminar, or (b) turbulent (Fig. 4.5). In (a), the flow pattern is not a square wave but axial streaming is present. In (b), turbulence has flattened the front and is making it less sharp. Both these effects tend to 'smear' the front along the airway. Turbulent eddies at the points of branching of the airways and the churning action of the heart exacerbate mixing of gas at the front. In addition, unequal pathway lengths – from respiratory surfaces of the lungs to lips – combine with regional differences in airways resistance and lung

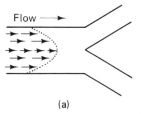 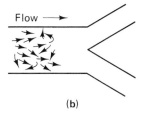

Fig. 4.5 Laminar (a) and turbulent (b) airflow in the trachea. With laminar flow the gas moves in organized layers parallel to the sides of the trachea, with peak velocity in the centre. Turbulent flow lacks this organization and the velocity profile is roughly square.

compliance to cause expired alveolar gas from different regions of the lungs to reach the lips at different times.

These considerations apply both to inspired and expired flows of gas, although it is convenient to consider the gas front as sharp and square, at least in quiet breathing. As the inspired air reaches the alveoli, it moves more by diffusion than by bulk flow, due to the rapid increase in total cross-sectional area of the airways. This slow-down of the advancing front allows concentration gradients to build up along the smaller airways. This *stratification* of incoming gas is less important in healthy lungs than in diseases in which the geometry of the small airways is changed to make the distances for diffusion unacceptably long; it may be important enough to restrict gas exchange. Similarly, the pathway length for diffusion is increased in alveoli whose airways become blocked and whose only ventilation is by collateral channels through pores in the walls of adjacent well-ventilated alveoli.

Inspired gas is not uniformly distributed, so at the end of inspiration alveolar gas is not of uniform composition throughout the lung, due to (1) differences in regional ventilation causing different dilutions of alveolar gas by inspired gas,

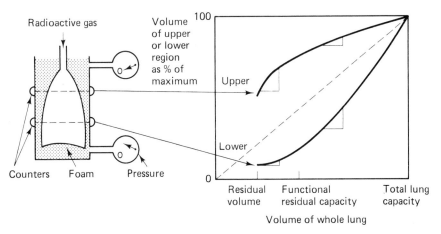

Fig. 4.6 The effect of a gradient of pressure due to gravity on regional ventilation. Ventilation is measured by counting the radioactivity over different regions of the chest when a radioactive tracer gas is inhaled. The graph shows the volumes of the upper and lower parts of the lungs (ordinate) as total lung volume (abscissa) increases from residual volume to total lung capacity. (See text for description.)

and (2) different blood flows exchanging O_2 and CO_2 with the alveolar gas at different rates. This is considered in Chapter 7.

Regional ventilation

By 'ventilation' we mean the amount of gas moved into and out of a region, irrespective of the initial volume of the region. Reasons for differences in regional ventilation become clear if we consider the distribution of a radioactive tracer gas used to inflate isolated lungs suspended in a gradient of pressure which mimics that found in the upright human chest, i.e. increasing by 0.025 kPa (0.25 cmH$_2$O) for every centimetre moved towards the base of the lungs (see Chapter 2). This can be achieved by placing the lungs in a foam of appropriate specific gravity. The amount of radioactive gas in a region at any time during the inflation can be measured by radioactivity counters placed over the surface of the lungs (Fig. 4.6). The ordinate of Fig. 4.6 gives the volumes of the upper and lower regions of the isolated lungs as percentages of their ultimate volume when fully inflated. The abscissa gives the volume of the whole lungs, i.e. that of all regions. If the lungs were free of any gradient of pressure, both the upper and lower regions would expand at the same rate, and the points representing their volumes would be along the same line, shown as a dotted line in Fig. 4.6. With a gradient of pressure applied over the lungs, the two regions behave differently. The slope of the lines in Fig. 4.6 represents proportionate change of volume: the steeper the slope, the greater the proportionate change. You can see the following.

1. The lower lobe starts at a smaller percentage of maximal volume because it is compressed by the greater external pressure.
2. It follows that the ventilatory capacity of the upper region is smaller than that of the lower, i.e. it operates in the range between 40 per cent and 100 per cent of its total volume range, while the lower lobe operates in the 15–100 per cent range. This is because the upper region is more inflated initially.
3. At volumes well below FRC there is proportionately more inflation of the upper regions (compare slopes of lines in Fig. 4.6). This is because at these volumes some of the airways to the lower lobes close and it takes a critical pressure to re-expand them.
4. At larger lung volumes the situation reverses and there is more ventilation of the lower region.

In deflation, the points in Fig. 4.6 representing the volumes of the two lung regions travel down the two curves, and the same considerations apply.

Some of these differences can be seen in the alveoli from the top and bottom of a partially inflated lung frozen *in situ* in the vertical position (Fig. 4.7).

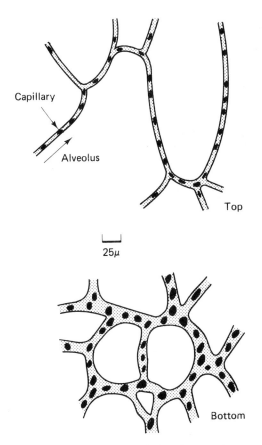

Fig. 4.7 Diagram of sections of a lung frozen in the vertical position. At the top the lung is relatively distended, and capillaries are empty of blood, compared with the situation at the bottom.

Measurement of uniformity of inspired gas distribution and mixing

Single breath washout curve

A single breath of O_2 is inspired and, during the following expiration, the N_2 concentration (F_{N_2}) (see Table 1.3 for 'F') at the mouth is measured (Fig. 4.8). In a healthy subject, N_2 in the expired air starts at zero (phase 1, dead space gas) and increases rapidly after the dead space is cleared (phase 2). It then continues to rise slightly (phase 3), due mainly to differences in ventilation of different lung regions. In disease, gross abnormalities of regional ventilation flatten phase 2 and introduce a conspicuous increase in F_{N_2} throughout phase 3. Careful examination of the normal curve shows a slight up-turn (phase 4) as the lung volume approaches RV. This is due to airway closure in the lower lobes causing a

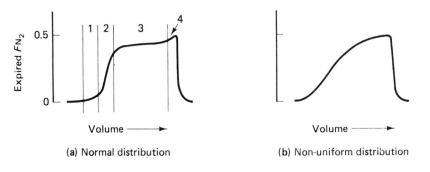

Fig. 4.8 Concentration of N_2 plotted against volume in a single expired breath after inhaling a breath of pure O_2. (a) The response of a healthy subject. The curve can be divided into four phases, which are described in the text. (b) A possible response from a patient with lung disease causing abnormalities of ventilation in different regions. The phases can no longer be clearly defined.

disproportionate amount of gas to come from the upper regions, which have a higher F_{N_2} (see Chapter 7). The lung volume at which the effect starts is called the critical closing volume (CCV). Diseases of the airways may accentuate phase 4 by causing airway closure at higher lung volume, and measurement of CCV is sometimes used as a test for airways disease.

Multiple breath washout curve

If, after breathing room air, a subject inhales continuously from a bag of pure O_2 and exhales through a N_2 meter, the concentration of N_2 in each breath is seen to fall due to the residual N_2 being 'washed out' of his lungs. This is the same process as repeatedly rinsing a piece of cloth which has been dyed; the colour of the water of each successive rinse becomes less and less. The concentration of N_2 (or dye) falls in an exponential curve. If we plot the log of concentration against the number of breaths of O_2 taken, the graph is nearly a straight line for healthy lungs with complete washout of N_2 in about 5–7 min (Fig. 4.9). In diseases with less uniform distribution of ventilation, the line becomes less steep and more non-linear, and the time for complete washout is prolonged.

Physiological factors influencing distribution

Breathing pattern and lung volume

Increased tidal volume and breathing rate have little effect on distribution. Reduced lung volume affects distribution if airway closure occurs.

Age

Distribution becomes increasingly non-uniform with age due to differences in the mechanical properties of lung regions with degenerative changes. In addition, the critical closing volume increases with age. This becomes very important

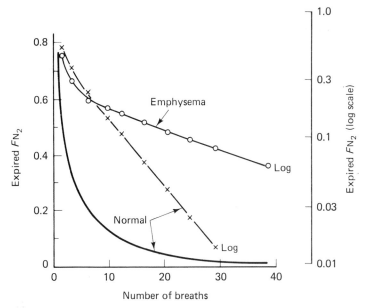

Fig. 4.9 Concentration of N_2 (F_{N_2}) in sequential expired breaths during breathing pure O_2. The thick line gives an actual example, while the crosses indicate the same values plotted with F_{N_2} on a log scale. Note that the latter is nearly linear. The circles are results for a patient with impaired uniformity of gas mixing in the lungs. In this case the log plot is very alinear and N_2 washout is far slower.

when some airways remain closed at FRC, or even throughout the whole of a normal breath, as it makes parts of the lungs ineffective at gas exchange.

Posture

Regional ventilation and perfusion patterns shift with posture due to the influence of gravity.

Airways smooth muscle tone

Histamine and other smooth muscle-contracting substances increase non-uniform distribution of ventilation by changing the mechanical properties of lung regions. Abolition of smooth muscle tone by drugs also reduces uniformity of distribution. This suggests that normal muscle tone minimizes non-uniform distribution.

Disease

Lung disease can produce gross inequalities of gas distribution, which are discussed in Cameron and Bateman (1983), Chapter 2.

Diffusion

We have followed the journey of inspired air through the bronchial tree to the respiratory surfaces of the alveoli, where diffusion equilibrates the gases in blood and air. The process of equilibration involves two very different states, the physics of which has been described in Chapter 1.

The gaseous state

In the alveoli, gas molecules move across the air space, to or away from the capillaries in the walls. The molecular weights of CO_2 and O_2 are 44 and 32 respectively, so from Graham's Law (see Chapter 1), CO_2 diffuses at 0.86 times the rate of O_2. This is close enough to unity to mean that CO_2 and O_2 diffuse with similar ease in the alveolar gas.

The liquid state

Once it has transversed the air spaces, a molecule of gas has to pass through a liquid and tissue layer to reach the blood in the capillaries. The rate of diffusion of a gas in a liquid across a membrane depends on Fick's Law, which has been described in Chapter 1. The rate depends not only on the pressure gradient but also on the solubility of the gas, and inversely as the square root of its molecular weight.

Once in solution, the rate of diffusion of a gas varies with its solubility. The solubilities of CO_2 and O_2 in tissue fluid are respectively 7.70 and 0.33 ml . ml^{-1} . kPa^{-1} (0.592 and 0.025 ml · ml^{-1} . mmHg^{-1}), a ratio of 23:1. Thus the solubilities of O_2 and CO_2 are more important than their molecular weights, and CO_2 passes from blood to alveolar air about twenty times more easily than O_2 passes in the opposite direction. If the alveolar wall is thickened and gas transfer is restricted, problems will arise with diffusion of O_2 well before CO_2 is significantly influenced. Nevertheless, in the whole lung equilibrium for CO_2 is established at about the same rate as that for O_2 because:

1. the reaction releasing CO_2 from blood is relatively slow;
2. the tension gradient driving CO_2 from blood to alveolus is only 0.8 kPa (6 mmHg), while that driving O_2 in the opposite direction is 8 kPa (60 mmHg) (see Chapter 5).

Time for diffusion

In normal lungs, blood takes about 1.0 s to pass through pulmonary capillaries, if the subject is at rest. This time is quite long enough for gaseous equilibrium to be established between the blood and alveolar gas. Even when the subject is exercising and the blood is flowing more quickly, there is adequate time for equilibration. Thus the blood leaving ventilated alveoli (end-capillary blood) has the same O_2 and CO_2 tensions as those in the alveoli it has just perfused.

Diffusing capacity

The alveolar wall is normally 0.1–0.5 μm thick. Any increase in thickness slows diffusion so that there may not be sufficient time for equilibration between alveolar gas and capillary blood. The same is true if the total diffusion area, normally 90 m³ in man, is decreased. To measure the lungs' ability to allow gas to pass from blood to alveoli (or vice versa), we measure their *diffusing capacity*, sometimes called the transfer factor:

$$\text{diffusing capacity} = \frac{\text{rate of gas transfer from lung to blood}}{\text{driving pressure (lung–blood)}}$$

Carbon monoxide (CO) is a convenient gas to use in the estimation of diffusing capacity. Provided that a low concentration is used its pressure in blood, where it combines avidly with haemoglobin (see page 70), is negligible. This makes the calculation of driving pressure, which will be the same as the alveolar tension of CO, fairly easy. The rate of CO transfer is the same as the rate of CO uptake by the lungs, and this is also quite easy to determine.

Diffusing capacity is reduced by thickening or by oedema of the alveolar capillary walls, by increased fluid lining the alveoli and by emphysematous changes which increase the distance for gaseous diffusion and decrease the alveolar capillary area available for diffusion. A decrease from the normal diffusing capacity for CO of about 6 ml . s · kPa⁻¹ (25 ml . min⁻¹ . mmHg⁻¹) occurs if the surface of the alveoli is reduced in area or increased in thickness, or if the distance over which respiratory gases have to diffuse between bronchioles and alveoli is increased in destructive diseases of the lungs.

Physiological changes in diffusion capacity are probably not very large, except in the case of exercise when previously closed capillaries open, there is an increase in the area for diffusion, and diffusing capacity increases by up to one-third.

Learning objectives

You should now be able to:

1. understand the importance of the structure of the respiratory tract to lung ventilation;
2. define anatomical and physiological dead spaces and describe how to measure them;
3. describe and explain normal differences in regional ventilation;
4. understand how to measure non-uniform distribution of ventilation;
5. explain the phases of a single breath N_2 washout curve;
6. describe the physiological factors influencing the distribution of ventilation;
7. describe the composition of alveolar gas and define respiratory exchange ratio;
8. describe how the processes of gas diffusion apply in the lungs;
9. define diffusing capacity.

5

PULMONARY CIRCULATION

For a region of the lung to operate efficiently, its ventilation should be matched by an appropriate blood supply, sufficient to carry away O_2 and to load the alveolar air with CO_2 for expiration. High blood flow should not be wasted on those regions with poor ventilation and with little to contribute to the arterialization of the blood. In this chapter the pulmonary circulation is described and some differences between it and the systemic circulations are discussed.

Blood flow in the lungs

The pulmonary circulation is sometimes called the 'lesser' circulation. This is a somewhat inappropriate term since the total lung blood flow almost equals the sum of the flows through all other organs of the body.

Pulmonary blood flow (right ventricular output) is not quite as large as cardiac output (left ventricular output) because:
1. the bronchial circulation, arising from the aorta, supplies the intrapulmonary airways and mainly drains into the pulmonary veins (Fig. 5.1);
2. the coronary circulation, also arising from the aorta, partly drains directly into the left ventricle via the Thebesian veins.
About 2 per cent of the total pulmonary arterial flow bypasses the respiratory surfaces and adds venous blood to the oxygenated blood returning to the left heart. This represents one form of 'shunt' which reduces the efficiency of the lungs.

Resistance to flow in the pulmonary circulation resides mainly in its arterioles and capillaries. It is normally about one-sixth of the total systemic vascular resistance; as a result of this and because their total blood flows are about the same, much lower pressures are developed in the pulmonary than in the systemic arteries. In pulmonary hypertension, in addition to the strain on the right heart, there is the threat that fluid forced from the lung capillaries by the high pressure within them will impair gas exchange or even obstruct the airways. To ensure that pulmonary capillary pressures are maintained low in conditions such as exercise, when cardiac output may increase five times or more, the pulmonary circulation has a remarkable ability to reduce its already low resistance. Open capillaries distend and closed capillaries open in response

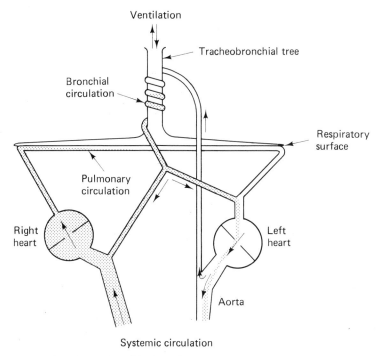

Ventilation

Tracheobronchial tree

Bronchial
circulation

Respiratory
surface

Pulmonary
circulation

Right
heart

Left
heart

Aorta

Systemic circulation

Fig. 5.1 The relationship of the bronchial circulation to the systemic and pulmonary circulations. Note how the bronchial circulation adds venous blood (shaded) to the arterialized blood in the left heart.

to increased perfusion pressure (Fig. 5.2). Pulmonary arterioles can also constrict, for example in response to hypoxia and various chemical mediators, and pulmonary hypertension is produced.

These vascular responses can take place in lungs which have been isolated from the body; they are therefore independent of the nervous system. They can occur in very localized regions of the lungs, and provide a mechanism for adjusting blood perfusion to match ventilation.

Blood flow through the pulmonary capillaries is much more pulsatile than flow through the systemic capillaries. This is firstly because arteriolar resistance is low and easily transmits pulsations, and secondly because capillaries in the upper parts of the lungs only open during systole and have no flow in diastole (see below). These pulsations are clearly demonstrated by the changes in pressure in an airtight container (a 'whole-body plethysmograph') inside which a subject inhales a highly soluble gas (e.g. N_2O) from a bag. As the gas dissolves in the blood in the lung capillaries, the alveolar and therefore total volume decreases causing a fall in pressure within the container. This fall in pressure is pulsatile, in step with the surges of blood through the lungs.

Only about one-sixth (75–100 ml) of the blood in the pulmonary circulation is in the pulmonary capillaries and takes part in gas exchange. The stroke volume of the heart at rest is about 70 ml, so nearly all the capillary blood is replaced at each

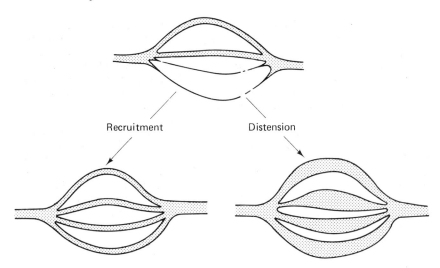

Fig. 5.2 The resistance of the pulmonary circulation can be reduced either by the recruitment of previously closed vessels, or by distension of previously open vessels, or both.

heart beat. Because the pulmonary arteries are distensible, the pulsations of blood flow in the capillaries are partly smoothed out.

Regional distribution of blood flow

Like inspired gas (see Chapter 4), blood flow is not uniformly distributed throughout the human lungs. Blood flow is greater in the base than in the apex of the upright lung. This difference is abolished when the subject lies down.

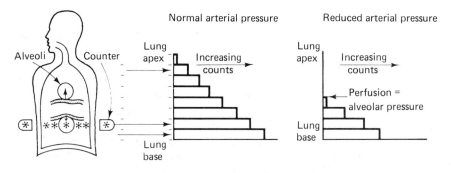

Fig. 5.3 Measurement of regional blood flow using radioactive xenon injected into the pulmonary circulation. The xenon in different parts of the lungs is measured by counters over the chest. The graph shows the relationship between blood flow and the level at which it is measured in an erect subject. On the right is shown what would happen to regional blood flow if pulmonary arterial pressure were allowed to fall, with the subject still erect. (After West 1976.)

Regional differences in blood flow can be measured by injecting into the pulmonary artery radioactive particles which are just too large to pass through the pulmonary capillaries. Most of the particles lodge where there is most blood flow, and radioactivity measured from outside the chest is proportional to regional flow. The procedure of deliberately blocking lung capillaries is not as dangerous as it sounds. Only a small proportion of capillaries need be occluded and the radioactive material is usually attached to albumen which is broken up in a few hours.

An alternative method of measuring regional blood flow (Fig. 5.3) is to inject ^{133}Xe (a radioactive gas) dissolved in saline into the right heart via an intravenous catheter. The gas leaves the blood by diffusion into the air of the alveoli. The subject holds his breath during the injection and the increase of radioactivity in a region of the lungs is proportional to blood flow in that region. The subject then re-breathes from a closed container and the radioactive gas becomes distributed throughout the lungs. If ventilation is uniform, the final distribution of radioactivity will correspond to the volumes of different regions of the lungs, and the blood flow per unit lung volume can be calculated.

Causes of uneven distribution of blood flow

If an isolated lung is suspended in a closed box where it can be ventilated by negative pressure and perfused with blood, the blood flow, measured by the methods described, increases from apex to base as in Fig. 5.3. As in any vascular bed, flow depends on the pressure difference between artery and vein and the resistance of the intervening vessels.

Blood flow through the lungs is a special case because they are filled with gas at a pressure uniformly close to atmospheric. Therefore the hydrostatic pressure of the blood within the capillaries has a greater distending effect at the base than at the apex of the lungs. If the alveoli were filled with a liquid of the same density as blood, the capillaries at the base of the lung would not be thus distended because their internal pressure would be exactly balanced by the external pressure due to the hydrostatic force of the liquid in the alveoli. This concept may be clearer if you refer to Fig. 5.4. The fact that the lungs contain air means there are three pressures we must consider when talking about blood flow in any region of the lung.

1. The *hydrostatic pressure* is determined by the distance of any region of the lung above the base. This hydrostatic pressure varies in the same way as pressure in any vertical column of liquid. It distends the vessels at the base of the lungs and allows those at the apex to be narrower, or even to collapse. Hydrostatic pressure is applied both to arteries and to veins; the pressures created by the right ventricle are superimposed on the arterial column of blood, and those created by the left atrium on the venous column.

2. The *difference in pressure* between the arterial and venous ends of lung capillaries drives blood through them. But blood only flows when the hydrostatic pressure (1. above) keeps the capillaries open.

3. *Alveolar air pressure.* The lung capillaries are separated from the alveoli by such a thin layer of tissue that the alveolar pressure, which is normally close to atmospheric, can act as a clamp and squeeze the capillaries shut if it is greater than capillary hydrostatic pressure. This can happen at the top of the lungs, especially if hydrostatic pressure is reduced, for example by haemorrhage.

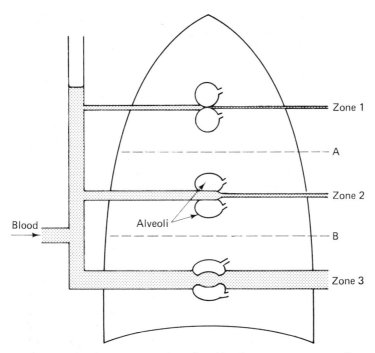

Fig. 5.4 How alveolar pressure and capillary blood pressure interact to influence blood flow in different regions of the upright lung. The three patterns of perfusion correspond to the three zones described in the text, where they are explained.

In fact pulmonary capillary blood pressure, especially near the top of the lung, is usually less than atmospheric or alveolar air pressure, because the blood vessels pass through the apex of the lung surrounded by intrapleural space where pressure is negative.

The interaction of these three pressures gives rise to three general zones of blood flow (Fig. 5.4).

Zone 1. If arterial pressure is less than alveolar pressure, which is usually near atmospheric, capillaries are collapsed and no flow takes place. This could occur *at the apex of the lungs* if there were pulmonary arterial hypotension, and would at first only occur in diastole.

Zone 2. Here, *lower in the lungs,* arterial pressure is high enough to hold the capillaries open. However, the pressure decreases along the capillaries, due to their resistance. Thus alveolar pressure is greater than venous pressure and the venules tend to collapse. This is a rather unstable condition with capillaries opening and closing, and flow rate depends on the difference between arterial and alveolar pressures. This is the mechanism of a 'Starling resistor', which is a collapsible tube (capillaries and venules) surrounded by a pressure chamber (alveoli).

Zone 3. Here, both arterial and venous pressures are always greater than alveolar pressure and they hold the capillaries open so that flow is continuous. The high venous pressure also helps to increase blood flow by distending the veins and venules, thereby reducing vascular resistance. This pattern is characteristic of the *base of the lungs.*

The three zones described for the excised lungs correspond in general with the regions of blood flow shown diagrammatically in Fig. 5.4, which represents the erect human lungs. They are not distinct, of course, but they gradually merge one into the other.

Pulmonary arterial systolic and diastolic pressures are on average about 3.5 and 1.3 kPa (28 and 10 mmHg). They would lift a column of blood about 35 and 13 cm above the heart respectively. The apex of the adult lung (which may act as for zone 1) is about 15 cm above the heart, so contractions of the right ventricle should pump blood through the apex in systole but not diastole. The intermittent apical flow may in part explain the pulsatile flow of the *whole* lung circulation mentioned above. Figure 5.3 shows what would happen to regional blood flow in an erect man if pulmonary arterial pressure fell.

In summary, flow at the top of the lung has the characteristics of zones 1 and 2. Lower down (below level A, Fig. 5.4) flow is that described for zone 2, where alveolar pressure (atmospheric) may be greater than venous pressure. At the base of the lung (below level B, Fig. 5.4) flow is as for zone 3, with both arterial and venous pressures above atmospheric.

An analogy may be drawn between the three types of blood flow and a crowd of people passing through swing doors fitted with very strong springs. If the pressure of the crowd (arterial pressure) is too low, they cannot force their way through the doors (no-flow zone 1). As the crowd builds up, people force their way through a few at a time but the doors slam shut after each group (pulsatile opening of capillaries). When the crowd is very large, their pressure holds the doors open and they pass through continuously (middle of lung zone 2). Finally, those who have already passed through can help to hold the doors open so that there is maximum flow (the effect of venous pressure at the bases of the lungs, zone 3).

Of course, this description is a simplification. Not all small vessels in the lung have the same surroundings, and conditions change during the respiratory cycle. Vessels in the alveolar walls are probably flattened as the alveoli expand during inspiration, and those between alveoli are elongated by a stretching action. These changes may explain why pulmonary vascular resistance increases during maximal lung inflation. In forced deflation, the capillaries may be compressed and kinked, again causing an increase in resistance.

Part of the pressure inside alveoli is dissipated in overcoming the surface tension of their liquid lining (see Chapter 2). This 'protects' the capillaries from some of the alveolar pressure and helps to keep them open.

Control of pulmonary blood flow

Blood flow in the lungs is mainly governed by the passive mechanisms we have outlined. Largely because of the paucity of smooth muscle in pulmonary arterioles, it was thought for many years that the pulmonary circulation had little or no vasomotor regulation. However, because pressure is low in the pulmonary arterioles, the tension in their walls is also low (Laplace's Law), and a little smooth muscle can easily adjust the radius. There is certainly sufficient smooth muscle in the arterioles to control the pulmonary circulation. This smooth muscle hypertrophies enormously in conditions such as chronic hypoxia and mitral valve disease when pulmonary pressures are high.

Local or systemic hypoxia is probably the most important physiological controller of pulmonary blood flow. Local hypoxic vasoconstriction directs blood away from poorly ventilated regions of the lungs. This mechanism can be demonstrated in isolated lungs and is therefore not a reflex. However, pulmonary arterioles separated from their surrounding tissue do not respond to hypoxia, which suggests that the lung parenchyma releases a vasoactive substance in response to low Po_2. A complementary mechanism exists in the airways, which are constricted by a fall in Pco_2 (see Chapter 3).

In experimental animals, systemic hypoxia, acting on peripheral chemoreceptors (see Chapter 8), reflexly constricts pulmonary arterioles, probably via the sympathetic nervous system. This could be a factor in the increased pulmonary arterial pressure which accompanies hypoxaemia of high altitude or disease.

Acetylcholine dilates constricted arterioles and used to be injected into the pulmonary circulation to determine what fraction of pulmonary hypertension is due to vasoconstriction as opposed to vascular obstruction. Breathing pure O_2-rich gas mixtures can also dilate pulmonary vessels, and this procedure is sometimes used in patients.

Learning objectives

You should now be able to:

1. describe the main structural and haemodynamic features of the pulmonary circulation and say how they differ from those of a systemic vascular bed;
2. explain why blood flow is not uniform throughout the lungs;
3. describe the mechanics of flow in each of the three 'zones' of the lung in an erect man;
4. know some chemical factors that control pulmonary vascular smooth muscle.

6

BLOOD GAS TRANSPORT AND pH

In blood, O_2 is carried mainly in combination with haemoglobin (Hb), with an insignificant amount in solution. Carbon dioxide is carried partly in solution, and partly in combination with proteins (in particular Hb), but mostly as bicarbonate. Changes in O_2 content affect CO_2 transport, and vice versa. Blood acidity depends on the responses of buffering systems, in particular protein, bicarbonate and phosphate, which take up hydrogen ions added to blood and release them again when the blood becomes more alkaline. Important values for normal blood are given in Table 6.1.

Table 6.1 Some values for normal blood.

		Systemic arterial blood	Mixed venous blood
Oxygen			
Tension	(mmHg)	100	40
	(kPa)	13.3	5.3
Blood content	(ml.litre^{-1})	200	150
Saturation	(%)	98	75
Carbon dioxide			
Tension	(mmHg)	40	46
	(kPa)	5.3	6.1
Blood content	(ml.litre^{-1})	490	530
Plasma content	(ml.litre^{-1})	600	640
Acidity			
Plasma [H$^+$]	(nM)	40	43
Plasma pH		7.40	7.37

Oxygen transport

Haemoglobin (Hb)

Haemoglobin consists of globin (a protein) and haem (a combination of ferrous iron and protoporphyrin). Every molecule of Hb contains four haem groups, each of which has a polypeptide chain, the four chains making up the globin. Haem has a constant chemical formula, but the polypeptide chains can vary and they determine the O_2-carrying characteristics of the blood; they are labelled with Greek letters, and the types of polypeptides present give the various forms of normal and abnormal Hb (see pages 68–70).

Normal adult human Hb has two alpha and two beta chains, with 141 and 146 amino acid residues per chain respectively; thus it has 574 amino acids which, with four haems, give a molecular weight of about 64 500. The analysis of the physical structure of the Hb molecule, and its relationship to O_2, is one of the most fascinating stories of modern biochemistry, but can only be touched on in this chapter (see Bartels and Bauman, 1977).

Combination of haemoglobin and oxygen

This is a reversible reaction:

$$Hb + O_2 \rightleftharpoons HbO_2 \qquad\qquad \textbf{6.1}$$

which will be driven to the right by an increase in Po_2 and vice versa. The Hb is deoxyhaemoglobin, often referred to as 'reduced haemoglobin', although the Hb is not chemically reduced. The HbO_2 is oxyhaemoglobin.

Each molecule of Hb contains four sites for combination with O_2, corresponding to the four haem groups and associated polypeptide chains (equation 6.1 should really be $Hb_4 + 4O_2 \rightleftharpoons Hb_4O_8$). The haem and globin groups in each molecule of Hb are held in a complex geometry by links ('salt-bridges') between the polypeptide chains. When a molecule of O_2 links to the iron atom in each haem, the molecular shape is distorted so that the attachment of the next O_2 molecule is easier. This allosteric effect explains the sigmoid shape of the graph of percentage saturation of Hb with O_2 plotted against Po_2 (Fig. 6.1a): the curvilinear relationship is the HbO_2 dissociation curve. When fully loaded, 1 g of Hb can carry about 2 mg, or 1.36 ml of O_2 at normal body temperature. Therefore 1 litre of normal blood, containing 150 g of Hb can transport about 200 ml of O_2 in HbO_2. This is the O_2 carrying capacity of the blood, or the volume of O_2 held in 1 litre of blood when the Hb is fully saturated.

There are a number of factors crucial to understanding O_2 transport by blood that relate to the HbO_2-dissociation curve and determine O_2 transport by the blood.

Oxygen tension (Po_2, kPa, mmHg)
This is sometimes called the partial pressure of the O_2 in solution. The Po_2 difference between two sites determines the direction and rate of flow of O_2. This is because the partial pressures correspond to concentrations *in solution* (see

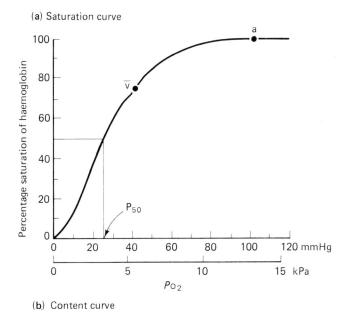

(a) Saturation curve

(b) Content curve

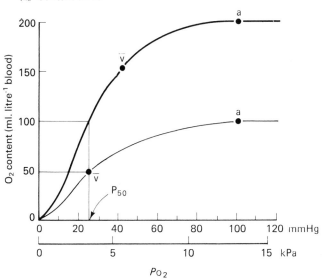

Fig. 6.1 (a) The oxyhaemoglobin-dissociation curve for adult Hb at pH 7.4 and temperature 37°C. The dissociation is expressed as percentage saturation and the P_{50} value is shown, typical values for arterial (a) and mixed venous (v̄) blood in a resting subject are given. The curve would be unchanged if the Hb content of blood was altered, although the v̄ point would be different.

(b) The same curve (thick line) as for (a) but with the ordinate giving O_2 content of blood rather than percentage saturation. The curve for blood containing only half the normal Hb (anaemia) is given (thin line). Note that both curves correspond to 100 per cent saturation at high PO_2s and that the P_{50}s are identical. The v̄ point is displaced downwards on the anaemic curve assuming that the tissues extract the same amount of O_2 for the same blood flows.

Chapter 1, Henry's Law), and dissolved O_2 will flow down its concentration gradient. Active skeletal muscle may have a Po_2 in the tissue of less than 1 kPa (7 mmHg). Arterial blood going to the muscle has a Po_2 of about 13 kPa (100 mmHg). The large pressure difference (12 kPa, 93 mmHg) strongly 'pushes' O_2 into the tissues. The rate at which the bloodstream can provide O_2 depends on the HbO_2 content and the blood flow to the tissues.

Haemoglobin content (Hb, g.litre^{-1}); oxygen content (ml.litre^{-1})
If blood is anaemic with (say) 50 per cent of normal Hb, then, even with complete saturation of Hb with O_2, a litre of blood only contains half the normal amount of O_2 (100 ml rather than 200 ml) (Fig. 6.1b). The O_2 content of blood, and its supply to the tissues, therefore depends both on Po_2 and on Hb content.

Haemoglobin saturation (percentage)
The *proportion* of the Hb combined with O_2 depends on Po_2 irrespective of the amount of Hb present. A Po_2 of 13 kPa (100 mmHg) produces virtually 100 per cent saturation. Measurement of Hb saturation is technically simple with spectrophotometry, which depends on the fact that HbO_2 is redder than Hb. Measurement of saturation is also convenient for clinical assessment since 100 per cent saturation in arterial blood implies full oxygenation and 'healthy' gas exchange. However, it gives less precise information about O_2 content and availability in the blood than do other measurements, particularly Po_2 and Hb content.

The oxyhaemoglobin (HbO_2) dissociation curve

The curve has already been described and illustrated (see Fig. 6.1). It can be expressed in two ways: as the relationship between Po_2 and *either* Hb saturation *or* O_2 content. Expressed as a Po_2/saturation relationship, the dissociation curve is independent of blood Hb content. However, the Po_2/content dissociation curve is displaced downwards in anaemia (where Hb content is low), indicating a smaller capacity of the blood to carry O_2 even when the Hb is fully saturated.

The shape of the HbO_2-dissociation curve has important physiological implications.

1. When Po_2 increases above about 10 kPa (70 mmHg), Hb does not take up much more O_2 because it is already nearly saturated; each molecule of Hb can carry only four molecules of O_2 however high the Po_2. Thus alveolar ventilation can decrease appreciably (by about 20–30 per cent) or increase indefinitely without the O_2 *content* of blood leaving the lungs varying significantly. The O_2 *tension* varies however. Therefore the large changes in ventilation seen in normal activities such as speech, sighing, emotion, coughing, etc., do not greatly change the amount of O_2 per unit of blood volume leaving the lungs and supplying the tissues.

2. As O_2 is withdrawn from the blood in response to a low Po_2 in active tissues, a small decrease in Po_2 or a small tension gradient delivering O_2 causes a large transfer of O_2, i.e. capillary blood works on the steep part of the HbO_2-dissociation curve. Thus, when tissues have a low Po_2 and therefore need much O_2, the HbO_2 can unload O_2 in large amounts. However, if there is decreased Hb

content in the blood (anaemia) and therefore less HbO_2, withdrawal of a little O_2 has a more profound effect; a low Po_2 and O_2 content are quickly reached with little further possible supply of O_2 to the tissues and a smaller Po_2 gradient to drive it in. Thus anaemia can cause tissue hypoxia although the arterial blood has a normal Po_2 and Hb saturation.

The position of the steep part of the HbO_2-dissociation curve is often expressed as its P_{50}, the Po_2 at which 50 per cent of the Hb is saturated. The P_{50} depends on the chemistry of the red cell contents, including the type of Hb present. The simplification of the curve to three points (origin, P_{50} and 100 per cent saturation) is valuable for a quick assessment of physiological and pathophysiological variations from normal blood. The P_{50} of normal adult human arterial blood is about 3.2 kPa (25 mmHg).

Factors that affect the oxyhaemoglobin dissociation curve

As already described, if the blood Hb is abnormal in amount, the curve is displaced up or down when the ordinate is expressed as O_2 content, but is unchanged when the ordinate is given as Hb saturation (see Fig. 6.1). The fact that in real life the Hb is concentrated in the special chemical environment of the red cell, rather than free in solution in plasma, is also a major factor in determining the precise HbO_2-dissociation curve (see below, DPG).

The position of the dissociation curve depends also on the chemical type(s) of Hb present both in physiological and pathological states (see pages 68–70).

Hydrogen ion concentration
Increased [H^+] (decreased pH, acidity) shifts the curve to the right, so that for a given Po_2 more O_2 will be released from HbO_2 (Fig. 6.2). This is called the *Bohr shift* and is due to H^+ acting on the Hb molecule to decrease its affinity for O_2, a reversal of the allosteric effect described earlier. In metabolizing tissues, release release of acids or of CO_2 (which increases [H^+]) thus liberates O_2 to flow down the O_2 pressure gradient and help fulfil the metabolic needs of the tissue. A decrease in pH of 0.2 units can increase O_2 release by 25 per cent at low Po_2s.

Carbon dioxide
Release of CO_2 from active tissues increases the [H^+] of the blood and shifts the curve to the right (Fig. 6.2); but in addition CO_2 reacts with Hb, forming carbamino-Hb (see below), and this also moves the curve to the right. If an increased Pco_2 (hypercapnia) is maintained for several hours, with chronic acidosis, red cell 2,3-diphosphoglycerate (DPG, see below) is decreased, shifting the curve back to the left.

Temperature
Increase in temperature dissociates HbO_2, i.e. shifts the curve to the right (Fig. 6.2). Thus blood gives up its O_2 less readily to cold tissues, so the blood leaving them may be well oxygenated because of this effect, and also because cold will lower the metabolic rate of tissues so that they require less O_2. This is why children playing in the snow usually have pink ears and noses when you might have expected their vasoconstricted skin to have turned blue. In the lungs, cold

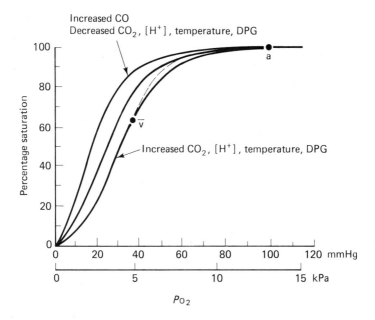

Fig. 6.2 The effect of $[H^+]$, CO_2, temperature, and 2,3-diphosphoglycerate on the HbO_2 dissociation curve. The effect of H^+ and CO_2 in moving the curve to the right is called the Bohr shift. The point for mixed venous blood ($\bar{v}$) in the resting subject will correspond to the right-hand curve so that the 'true' dissociation curve is represented by the interrupted line.

will, if anything, increase oxygenation of Hb by shifting the dissociation curve to the left. Although this effect is not normally important, it becomes so in patients who are made hypothermic during open heart surgery; in such patients even if the arterial Po_2 is low the Hb is relatively saturated and the patient does not look hypoxic.

2,3-Diphosphoglycerate (DPG)
In anaerobic glycolysis, most cells convert 1,3-diphosphoglycerate to 3-phosphoglycerate with release of energy to form adenosine triphosphate (ATP). Red cells are unusual in that they convert 1,3-DPG to 2,3-DPG with no formation of ATP (Fig. 6.3). However, the DPG reacts with HbO_2 which releases O_2, i.e. the dissociation curve shifts to the right (see Fig. 6.2). The importance of DPG in red cells can be seen in several situations.

1. In chronic hypoxia, due to disease or residence at high altitude, DPG increases so O_2 is more readily released in the hypoxic tissues. The effect may partly be due to decreased Pco_2 (hypocapnia), which increases DPG (the converse of the chronic effect of hypercapnia and acidosis mentioned above): CO_2 and DPG probably act at the same binding sites of the Hb molecule. Hyperoxia has the opposite effect to hypoxia on DPG concentration and on the HbO_2-dissociation curve.

2. In prolonged exercise, DPG increases, presumably because of the hypoxia, especially in venous blood, again shifting the curve to the right.

3. In stored blood, DPG content decreases and such blood, when transfused,

will not give up its O_2 readily. It can be treated to increase the DPG content.
4. Red cells with abnormal haemoglobins, e.g. those in sickle cell anaemia, may have more DPG than normal (see also fetal Hb, below).
5. The DPG content may be affected by enzyme abnormalities in red cells. Pyruvate kinase deficiency increases DPG, while hexokinase deficiency decreases it (Fig. 6.3).

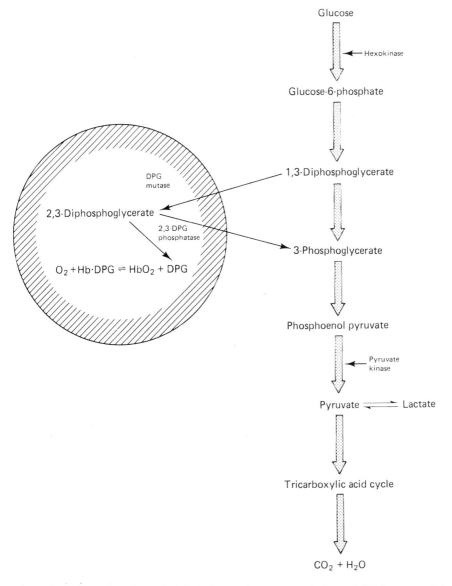

Fig. 6.3 The glycolytic pathway (right) which provides energy in the form of ATP for most cells is also present in erythrocytes. However, they have an extra 'shunt' (left) that produces 2,3-DPG and dissociates HbO_2.

In summary, the association and dissociation of Hb with O_2 normally maintain full oxygenation of arterial blood on the upper flat part of the dissociation curve, while the steep part of the curve allows release of large amounts of O_2 in active tissues. In the tissues, displacements of the curve to the right by H^+, P_{CO_2} and increased temperature promote greater release of O_2. In a rapidly metabolizing tissue, such as exercising muscle, the shift to the right is considerable and O_2 becomes much more readily available. Slower adjustments to the position of the dissociation curve may take place via DPG.

Note that a shift of the oxyhaemoglobin dissociation curve to the right as blood passes through actively metabolizing tissues in effect steepens the 'true' dissociation curve, the line that joins the arterial and venous points on the curves (see Fig. 6.2).

In healthy lungs, because HbO_2-dissociation curves under most conditions merge in the flat, fully saturated part, these physiological shifts do not hinder the loading of blood with O_2.

Why red blood cells?

The advantages of confining the Hb into red cells are as follows.

1. The chemical environment in the cell, especially the presence of DPG, displaces the dissociation curve to the right so that O_2 unloads readily in active tissues.
2. If 10 g of Hb were free in each litre of plasma, the viscosity of the blood would rise to intolerable values, and colloid osmotic pressure would also increase considerably. The viscosity effect is especially important in capillaries where the presence of red cells in blood gives it an anomalously low viscosity (the Fahraeus-Lindquist effect), although this effect is still open to dispute.
3. Hb molecules free in the plasma are just small enough to escape from the blood through the glomeruli of the kidneys and thus to be lost in the urine.
4. There are enzyme systems in the red cell which help prevent Hb breakdown; for example methaemoglobin reductase converts ferric methaemoglobin back to ferrous haemoglobin.
5. Carbonic anhydrase is restricted to the red cells and is crucial for the importance of the red cell in CO_2 transport.

Other forms of haemoglobin and their reactions

Fetal haemoglobin

The fetus has a haemoglobin with a high affinity for O_2, and this facilitates O_2 transfer from the mother to the fetus. Fetal Hb has two gamma-polypeptide chains in place of the beta-chains of adult Hb. Inside red cells, fetal Hb has a greater affinity for O_2 than does adult Hb (Fig. 6.4), probably because DPG is less active. In the uterine/placental circulation, where the P_{O_2} is lower than in maternal arterial blood, the fetal blood takes up O_2 mainly because the umbilical (fetal) arterial blood is more hypoxic than the maternal uterine arterial blood. In

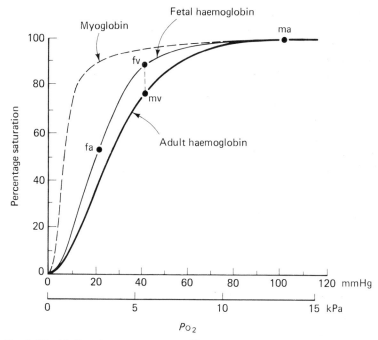

Fig. 6.4 The HbO$_2$ dissociation curves of fetal and adult blood. Points for maternal arterial (ma) and venous (mv) blood, and for fetal umbilical arterial (fa) and venous (fv) blood are given. The curve for myoglobin is also given (interrupted line).

addition, however, because the fetal Hb curve is to the left of the maternal one, when arterial blood from the maternal circulation equilibrates with umbilical blood, the fetal blood has a higher content of O$_2$ than has maternal blood. Thus when the PO$_2$ has equilibrated, the fetal blood is far more saturated with O$_2$ than is the maternal blood. An additional mechanism aiding transfer of O$_2$ from mother to fetus is that the unloading of CO$_2$ from fetal to maternal blood shifts the fetal dissociation curve to the left and the maternal curve to the right. This double Bohr shift, widening the gap between the two dissociation curves, further shifts the balance of O$_2$ towards the fetus.

This increased O$_2$ uptake and supply to the fetus is at the cost of a greater difficulty in releasing O$_2$ from blood in the fetal tissues which results in a degree of hypoxia; fetal tissues seem better able to withstand hypoxia than those in the adult. Fetal Hb is relatively more acid than adult Hb, and carries CO$_2$ less readily, so the fetus tends towards acidosis.

Fetal red cells contain a mixture of fetal and adult Hb, the former disappearing during the first few months after birth.

Myoglobin

This is a combination of one molecule of haem and one polypeptide chain, and occurs in skeletal and cardiac muscle fibres. Its dissociation curve is well to the left of that of Hb (Fig. 6.4), so it readily takes up O$_2$ from capillary blood.

Myoglobin may act as a small store of O_2 to be available in anaerobic conditions. When a muscle such as the heart contracts, its blood flow virtually ceases, but myoglobin can still release its O_2. When the muscle relaxes and the blood flow is re-established, myoglobin recharges with O_2. When blood flow to muscle is prevented, the myoglobin oxygen store is depleted in a few seconds.

Carboxyhaemoglobin (HbCO)

Carbon monoxide has 210 times greater affinity for Hb than does O_2. Since air contains about 21 per cent O_2, addition of 0.1 per cent CO leads to arterial blood having 50 per cent HbO_2 and 50 per cent HbCO, the equivalent to a 50 per cent anaemia; of course it takes quite a long time, over an hour, for enough CO at this concentration to be supplied to the blood to reach this equilibrium but, once there, CO takes an equally long time to be cleared from the blood. Ventilation with pure O_2 will speed elimination of CO, because at a high Po_2 O_2 competes more effectively for the binding sites on Hb.

Carbon monoxide in addition shifts the HbO_2 dissociation curve to the left (see Fig. 6.2), so that the 'anaemic' blood less readily gives up its O_2 in the tissues. The HbCO is cherry-red in colour, so patients poisoned by CO often look deceptively pink and healthy.

Methaemoglobin (Met-Hb)

Methaemoglobin is formed when the ferrous atom in Hb is oxidized to the ferric form. This can occur congenitally or in response to oxidizing poisons such as nitrites. The Met-Hb cannot combine with O_2. Red cells contain methaemo-globin reductase that converts Met-Hb back to Hb, but this enzyme is not present in plasma.

Abnormal haemoglobins

Well over a hundred different human Hbs with variants of the peptide patterns in the four polypeptide chains have been identified. Some of the Hbs have abnormal dissociation curves, either because of the Hb itself or because it leads to other changes in the red cell such as abnormal DPG content. Abnormalities of Hb may also change the shape of the red cell and make it more fragile, for example in sickle-cell anaemia.

Cyanosis

The colour of blood depends on the content of Hb and on the proportions of HbO_2 (red) and deoxy-Hb (purple). The skin will appear bluish (*cyanosis*) when the capillary blood in it contains about 50 g.litre^{-1} of deoxy-Hb. With normal blood this corresponds to about 70 per cent saturation and a Po_2 of 5 kPa (40 mmHg). In anaemia the percentage saturation has to be much lower to provide the same absolute amount of deoxy-Hb

The relationship between subjective appearance of cyanosis and the objective blood contents of Hb and HbO_2 is debatable, but the general conclusion is valid. Thus anaemic patients can be severely hypoxic without cyanosis and polycythaemic patients with excess Hb may be cyanosed with little hypoxia.

Oxygen in solution

The only way O_2 can travel to and from the red cell is in solution in plasma and tissue fluid. However, it is poorly soluble in these liquids. The amount in solution is directly proportional to the gas pressure (Henry's Law): 1 litre of normal arterial blood at a Po_2 of 13 kPa (100 mmHg) contains only 3 ml of O_2 in solution; 3 ml is one-sixtieth of the O_2 combined with Hb, and quantitatively of no importance. However, if a subject breathes pure O_2, the alveolar and arterial Po_2s will increase over sixfold, and the O_2 in solution will be about 20 ml per litre of blood. Although this is only one-tenth of the *total* O_2 combined with Hb, it is about two-fifths of that normally extracted from the blood, since mixed venous blood is 75 per cent saturated with O_2 (arteriovenous O_2-content difference, 50 ml per litre of blood). If a subject breathes pure O_2 at 3 atmospheres pressure, he can in theory obtain all the O_2 he needs from its solution in plasma, and Hb as an O_2 transporter becomes unnecessary.

Carbon dioxide transport

Nearly all the CO_2 in the blood usually comes from metabolizing tissues, where the gas in solution follows its pressure gradients from cell interior, to extracellular fluid, to plasma and red cell, to alveolar gas and finally to the outside air. Carbon dioxide is found in solution, in chemical combination to form HCO_3^-, and combined with amino groups of proteins, and there are also very small amounts of carbonic acid (H_2CO_3) and carbonate ion (CO_3^{2-}).

Plasma carbon dioxide

Dissolved CO_2 reacts with water to form HCO_3^- and H^+:

$$CO_2 + H_2O \rightleftharpoons H_2CO_3 \rightleftharpoons HCO_3^- + H^+ \qquad 6.2$$

In plasma the first stage is a slow reaction, and it takes 100 s to reach 90 per cent equilibrium at body temperature. Buffers such as plasma proteins take up most of the H^+, so $[H^+]$-changes are minimized.

Carbon dioxide also reacts with amino groups on plasma proteins to form carbamino compounds:

$$R\text{-}NH_2 + CO_2 \rightleftharpoons R\text{-}NHCOO^- + H^+ \qquad 6.3$$

and again H^+ is buffered.

Blood carbon dioxide

Because reaction 6.2 is slow, and reaction 6.3 is rather limited, CO_2 added to whole blood will at first increase the plasma Pco_2 appreciably, and CO_2 will

At the tissues

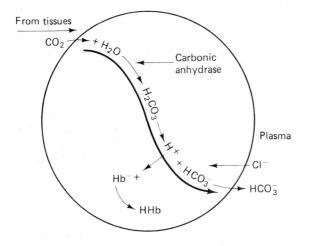

At the lungs

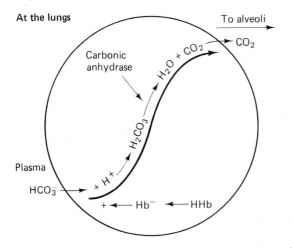

Fig. 6.5 How carbonic anhydrase in the red cells accelerates loading and unloading of plasma with CO_2 in the form of HCO_3. Note the Cl^- shift.

diffuse into the red cells. Here, both reactions 6.2 and 6.3 also occur, but with important differences. The enzyme *carbonic anhydrase* catalyses the formation of H_2CO_3 from CO_2 and H_2O. This enzyme is absent from the plasma. Thus in the red cell equation 6.2 goes quickly to the right, so that $[HCO_3^-]$ and $[H^+]$ increase. Both these ions are then removed, shifting equation 6.2 further to the right: H^+ is taken up by Hb, and HCO_3^- diffuses into the plasma along its concentration gradient. The chloride ion enters the red cell from the plasma so that electrical neutralities in the cell and plasma are maintained. This movement of ions is called the *chloride shift* (Fig. 6.5), and if it did not take place HCO_3^- would be held in the red cell and less CO_2 could be converted to HCO_3^-.

The proteins with which reaction 6.3 takes place include haemoglobin. Haemoglobin is quantitatively more important than plasma protein because normal blood contains four times as much Hb as plasma protein, and because, for equal quantities, Hb has three-times greater affinity for CO_2 than do plasma proteins. The Hb combines with CO_2, to form carbamino-Hb, according to the reaction:

$$Hb\text{-}NH_2 + CO_2 \rightleftharpoons Hb\text{-}NHCOO^- + H^+ \qquad\qquad 6.4$$

The H^+ formed in red cell from equations 6.2 and 6.4 is buffered by Hb. Deoxygenated Hb is a weaker acid than HbO_2 and has more sites available to take up H^+; it therefore absorbs more H^+ and equation 6.4 shifts to the right. In other words, the release of O_2 from HbO_2 into active tissues allows the Hb to take up and carry more CO_2 for the same PCO_2.

Changes at the lungs

In the lungs the reverse processes take place to those in the tissues (Fig. 6.5). As CO_2 is blown-off, equations 6.2, 6.3 and 6.4 move to the left, and the chloride shift is reversed. The oxygenation of Hb to HbO_2 moves equation 6.4 to the left,

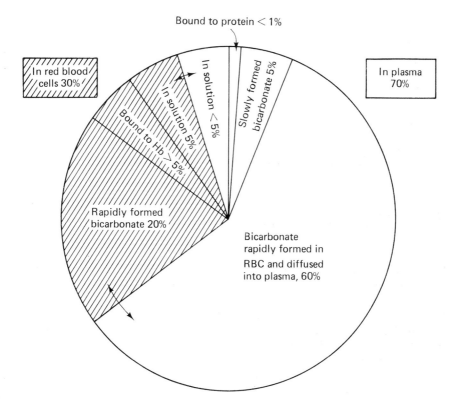

Fig. 6.6 The forms in which CO_2 is carried in the red cells and plasma.

since HbO_2 binds CO_2 less strongly than does deoxy-Hb, and HbO_2 is a stronger acid than is deoxy-Hb. These changes aid the release of CO_2 from the red cell into the plasma and alveoli.

Transport of carbon dioxide

The quantities of the main forms of transported CO_2 are shown in Fig. 6.6 and Table 6.1. However, although the total *amount* of CO_2 carried in red cells is considerably less than that carried in plasma, the chemical reactions of CO_2 in the red cells with subsequent buffering of the H^+ produced are greater than in the plasma. Thus the *exchange* of CO_2 in tissues and lungs depends more on the red cells than on the plasma contents. This fact can be shown by inhibiting the carbonic anhydrase in the red cells by a suitable drug; now CO_2 entering the blood is only slowly converted to HCO_3^-, so the amounts in solution and as plasma carbamino compounds build up with resultant acidosis.

Carbon dioxide dissociation curve

The amount of CO_2 in solution in blood or tissue fluid depends on the tension (partial pressure) of the gas in contact with that solution (Henry's Law). The P_{CO_2} therefore determines the degree of formation of HCO_3^- and carbamino compounds by equations 6.2, 6.3 and 6.4. The relationship between P_{CO_2} and *total* CO_2 in blood (or plasma) is the CO_2-dissociation curve (Fig. 6.7). It is approximately linear over the physiological range of P_{CO_2}s from mixed venous to arterial blood, 6.0–5.2 kPa (46–40 mmHg). Since HbO_2 has a weaker affinity for CO_2 than has deoxy-Hb, oxygenated blood has a curve displaced to the right (the Haldane shift); HbO_2 is a stronger acid than is deoxy-Hb and releases H^+ which helps to reverse equations 6.2 and 6.4. The result is that the 'true' physiological CO_2-dissociation curve is steeper than might be expected, since it joins the a and v̄ points on Fig. 6.7; in other words, at any P_{CO_2} blood loads and unloads extra CO_2 when O_2 is also unloaded and loaded.

Note that the CO_2-dissociation curve cannot be 'saturated', unlike the combination of Hb and O_2. Although normally Hb content (150g.litre^{-1}) and therefore O_2 capacity of blood (200 ml.litre^{-1}) are fairly constant, the CO_2 content of blood is quite variable even in health.

Combined oxygen and carbon dioxide transport in blood

At rest, our tissues utilize about 250 ml.min^{-1} of O_2 and produce about 200 ml.min^{-1} of CO_2. Normal cardiac output is about 5 litres.min^{-1}. If you look at the dissociation curves for HbO_2 and CO_2, you will see that removing 250 ml of O_2 from 5 litres of blood will reduce the P_{O_2} by about 8 kPa (60 mmHg), while adding 200 ml of CO_2 to 5 litres of blood will increase the P_{CO_2} by about 0.8 kPa (6 mmHg). Thus the combined tensions of CO_2 and O_2 will be about 7 kPa (50 mmHg) less in mixed venous than in arterial blood (see Table 6.1, page 61). If there is a pocket of air at atmospheric pressure in the tissues, the proportions of O_2, CO_2 and N_2 will first move towards those corresponding to the tensions of the

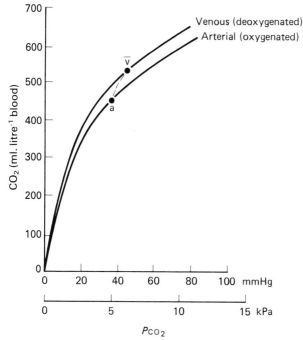

Fig. 6.7 The amount of CO_2 carried by whole blood at different $P\text{co}_2$s (the CO_2 dissociation curve) is influenced by the degree of oxygenation of the blood. The two curves represent the levels of oxygenation found in arterial and venous blood. The points a and $\bar{v}$ represent the CO_2 contents and tensions of normal arterial and mixed venous blood for a resting subject. The 'true' CO_2 dissociation curve over the range found in the body is represented by the interrupted line joining a and $\bar{v}$. Note that $P\bar{v}\text{co}_2$ is about 0.5 kPa (4 mmHg) lower than it would be if the blood remained oxygenated. This Haldane effect helps the tissues unload their CO_2 into the blood.

gases in capillary blood; in particular, O_2 will be taken up and CO_2 given off by the blood. Then, since end-capillary blood always has a total gas tension less than atmospheric pressure, all three gases will have tension gradients that absorb them into the blood. This result is entirely due to the shape of the two dissociation curves. It can be speeded up by giving the subject pure O_2 to breathe since the arterial blood has N_2 displaced from it by O_2 (with high $Pa\text{o}_2$), while capillary blood has both a low $P\text{N}_2$ and a low $P\text{o}_2$, reducing the total gas tension even more.

Acid-base balance

Acids are being continually formed in the body by oxidation of proteins and nucleic acids (producing sulphuric and phosphoric acids), conversion of metabolic CO_2 to carbonic acid, and release of lactic and other acids in anaerobic metabolism of carbohydrate and fat, for example in exercise. (Oxygen means 'acid producer' in Greek.) These acids dissociate (ionize) to increase the $[H^+]$ (H^+ concentration) of the blood. (Acids, by definition, are proton donors. In aqueous solution they increase $[H^+]$ and the H^+ combines with H_2O to form H_3O^+, but it is conventional to speak of hydrogen ions.) The blood buffer systems neutralize most of this excess H^+, but this only gives a respite to the problem. In the long term the body must rid itself of as much acid as it produces.

Carbon dioxide is excreted in the lungs, the H^+ which it had formed being converted back to water (reversal of equation 6.2). Non-volatile acids are excreted by the kidneys, in particular as sulphate and phosphoric acids. The normal pH of the urine is about 6.0, showing that the body is producing an excess of acid over that removed in respiration.

Strictly speaking, the lungs do not 'excrete acid'. They excrete CO_2 which, if allowed to remain in the body, would produce acidaemia. When acids such as lactic are added to the blood, they displace equation 6.2 to the left, forming CO_2 and water. The removal of this CO_2 in the lungs limits the acidosis which would otherwise be more severe.

The total amount of non-volatile acids produced each day by a normal healthy man exceeds 50 mmol and this has to be disposed of. Also about 12 mol CO_2 (250 times as much 'acid') is produced each day. If acids formed by metabolism did not ionize in solution in body fluids and could be excreted as such by the kidney, there would be little problem; however, the only metabolic acids which do not ionize strongly are monobasic phosphoric acid, β-hydroxybutyric acid and creatinine. All the others are almost completely ionized and so create the physiological problem of controlling blood and urine $[H^+]$. Urine never has a pH below about 4.5. Even although some additional H^+ can be buffered by ammonia secreted in the kidney, the power of the kidney to eliminate acid is severely limited. When you consider the relative amounts of acid disposed of by the lungs and by the kidneys, you will understand why some respiratory physiologists imply that the kidneys are mere extensions of the lungs.

Body compartments

In this book we consider acid-base balance only in relation to the blood. However, this is only one of the three body fluid compartments (blood, interstitial fluid and intracellular fluid) and, in terms of *total* CO_2, H^+ and HCO_3^- contents, of least importance. The blood system is also unique in its dynamic nature, moving from tissues to lungs where acid-base conditions are very different. In respiratory physiology it is convenient to consider blood acid-base balance in isolation, but in clinical physiology the interactions between the three compartments are of great importance. They are considered in detail in Cameron and Bateman (1983), Chapter 8. It may be noted that the same general consideration does not apply to O_2 balance because, although Po_2 gradients in the tissues and O_2-binding substances such as myoglobin in cells are important, blood contains almost all the total body O_2 due to its Hb.

Normal blood hydrogen ion concentration

Normal plasma $[H^+] = 40$ nmol (pH $= 7.40$). An increase or a decrease causes, respectively, acidaemia or alkalaemia, which can be physiological or pathological. Because the pH scale is logarithmic, a shift of one unit represents a tenfold change in $[H^+]$. Addition or removal of H^+ to the blood activates blood buffering, changes in respiratory excretion of CO_2 and changes in renal excretion of H^+ and HCO_3^-.

Blood buffering

A *strong* acid is one that dissociates to a large extent in solution; strong in this chemical sense does not mean concentrated. Buffers are solutions that resist changes in $[H^+]$ when acids or bases are added to them. Buffers consist of weak acid $[H^+A^-]$, one that only slightly dissociates into H^+ and anion, and its salt that dissociates more freely. In an aqueous solution of the two the following reaction is set up with the equilibrium well to the left:

$$H^+A^- + A^- + Na^+ \rightleftharpoons A^- + H^+ + Na^+A^- \qquad \textbf{6.5}$$

where A^- is the anion. Addition of a strong acid, such as H^+Cl^-, will shift the reaction further to the left because of the strong affinity of A^- for the added H^+. Thus the potential increase in H^+ is minimized. The added Cl^- associates with Na^+ to form neutral Na^+Cl^-.

An important aspect of buffering action is the pK of the system. This is determined by measuring the degree of dissociation of the acid at different pHs. The pK is the pH at which the buffer salt and the acid are each half-dissociated, and therefore most effective as a buffer, i.e. the addition or removal of H^+ will cause the least change in pH. At pH values away from pK, the buffer system will be less effective, and addition or removal of H^+ will cause larger changes in pH. Since normal plasma pH is 7.40, a buffer system with a pK of this value will be

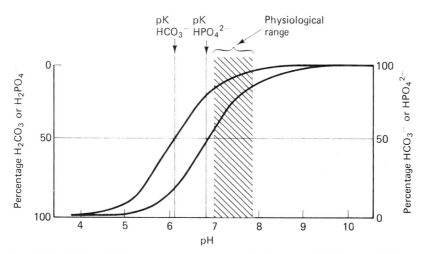

Fig. 6.8 The HCO_3^-/H_2CO_3 system is a most efficient buffer at its pK (6.1). At this pH the curve is steepest, so a change of HCO_3^-/H_2CO_3 proportions will cause least effect on pH. At the normal blood pH (7.40) the system is less efficient. The buffer system would be more efficient in urine which has on average a pH of about 6.0.

The $HPO_4^{2-}/H_2PO_4^-$ buffer system has a pK of 6.8 which is closer to the blood pH.

most powerful. Figure 6.8 illustrates graphically two buffer systems, for phosphate and for HCO_3^-. These buffer systems are found in blood, intracellular and interstitial fluids, urine and other body fluids, where their efficiency depends on pH which may be far from 7.40.

The main buffering systems in blood are bicarbonate, proteins including haemoglobin, and phosphate.

Protein buffers

Haemoglobin and plasma proteins constitute quantitatively the main blood systems for buffering added acid. Haemoglobin is more important than plasma proteins, partly because molecule-for-molecule it is a more efficient buffer, and also because it has a higher concentration in whole blood (150 g. litre^{-1} blood for Hb compared with 40 g. litre^{-1} blood for plasma proteins). Buffering action of protein is based on equation 6.3, where R- can be plasma proteins or Hb.

Bicarbonate buffer

The basic buffer equation for this system depends on the dissociation of carbonic acid in solution:

$$H_2CO_3 \rightleftharpoons H^+ + HCO_3^- \qquad\qquad 6.6$$

Addition of H^+ will shift the reaction to the left and H^+ will be taken up with little change in pH. Removal of H^+ shifts the reaction to the right producing more H^+ and again minimizing the change in pH.

The Law of Mass Action applied to equation 6.6 states that:

$$\frac{[H^+][HCO_3^-]}{[H_2CO_3]} = K_A \qquad\qquad 6.7$$

where K_A is the dissociation constant of H_2CO_3. Equation 6.7 can be converted to a special equation relevant to CO_2 carriage in blood, the *Henderson-Hasselbalch equation*.

Since pH is the negative logarithm of $[H^+]$, taking the log of both sides of equation 6.7 and transposing we get:

$$\log\frac{[H^+][HCO_3^-]}{[H_2CO_3]} = \log K_A \qquad\qquad 6.8$$

$$\log[H^+] + \log\frac{[HCO_3^-]}{[H_2CO_3]} = \log K_A \qquad\qquad 6.9$$

$$\log[H^+] = \log K_A - \log\frac{[HCO_3^-]}{[H_2CO_3]} \qquad\qquad 6.10$$

and since pH and pK_A are the negative logarithms of $[H^+]$ and K_A, respectively:

$$pH = pK_A + \log\frac{[HCO_3^-]}{[H_2CO_3]} \qquad\qquad 6.11$$

This is not a very useful equation because $[H_2CO_3]$ has such a small concentration in blood that it is not practical to measure it.

But since carbonic anhydrase (C.A.) in the red cells catalyses the reaction

$$CO_2 + H_2O \underset{}{\overset{\text{C.A.}}{\rightleftharpoons}} H_2CO_3$$

rapidly to equilibrium, addition of H^+ to whole blood shifts the reaction far to the left; at equilibrium, $[CO_2] = 809\,[H_2CO_3]$. Thus for whole blood, equation 6.11 can be written:

$$pH = pK' + \log \frac{[HCO_3{}^-]}{[CO_2]} \qquad \qquad \textbf{6.12}$$

Since $[CO_2]$ is proportional to P_{CO_2} (Henry's Law), we have the usual expression of the Henderson-Hasselbalch equation:

$$pH = pK' + \log \frac{[HCO_3{}^-]}{\alpha P_{CO_2}} \qquad \qquad \textbf{6.13}$$

where α is the solubility of CO_2 in plasma per kPa P_{CO_2} at 38°C (0.23 mmol . kPa^{-1}. litre^{-1} or 0.0310 mmol . mmHg^{-1}. litre^{-1}). The P_{CO_2} is relatively easy to measure with a 'CO_2-electrode'.

When we consider the CO_2-$HCO_3{}^-$ system as a buffer in whole blood, surprisingly its pK is 6.1 (see Fig. 6.6), far from the normal blood pH of 7.40; the $HCO_3{}^-$ buffer is about twenty times less efficient than if its pK were 7.40. In addition, this buffering action only works when non-volatile acids are added to blood or when CO_2 acts on proteins to release H^+.

The $HCO_3{}^-$ system is *not* a buffer *for* CO_2.
Remember:

$$CO_2 + H_2O \rightleftharpoons H_2CO_3 \rightleftharpoons H^+ + HCO_3{}^- \qquad \qquad \textbf{6.2}$$

and the reaction reaches equilibrium to the right, $[HCO_3{}^-]$ being twenty times greater than $[CO_2]$. Every molecule of CO_2 taking part in this whole reaction forms an H^+ and a $HCO_3{}^-$ ion, and this is *not* a buffering action. However, the system is essential for the *transport* of CO_2 (converted mainly to $HCO_3{}^-$) in blood. Without the reaction and its catalysis by carbonic anhydrase in the red cell, CO_2 would have to remain mainly in physical solution with very high P_{CO_2}s. (This happens when inhibitors of carbonic anhydrase are given.) In turn, the high P_{CO_2} would lead to H^+ release from proteins including haemoglobin. Thus the $HCO_3{}^-$ transport system and the rapid excretion of CO_2 by the lungs are essential for minimizing the acidaemia that results from the addition of CO_2 to the blood.

The ability of the blood system to *transport* CO_2 makes up for its weakness as a buffer. By transporting blood containing CO_2 and $HCO_3{}^-$ to the lungs and kidneys, it 'enlists their aid' in controlling the levels of these substances and therefore pH. The lungs excrete or retain CO_2 and the kidneys eliminate or retain $HCO_3{}^-$, and so both very efficiently maintain the $HCO_3{}^-$: CO_2 ratio at

20:1. Although not a buffer system, the kidney – HCO_3^- : CO_2 – lung combination is a more powerful determinant of blood pH than an excellent buffer such as Hb. The ability of Hb to deal with excess acid or base is limited by the amount of Hb present. The kidneys and lungs, on the other hand, can deal with an almost infinite excess of these substances because they simply pass them to the outside.

An analogy may be drawn with a man in a leaky rowing boat. He is far worse off with a large supply of the best quality sponges to mop up water which he is not allowed to wring out, than he would be with an efficient pump which ejects the encroaching water.

We should therefore modify the denigration of the kidneys as 'mere extensions of the lungs' (see page 76) to regard them as full partners in the regulation of the HCO_3^- : CO_2 ratio and therefore of pH. Indeed, the Henderson-Hasselbalch equation is sometimes qualitatively written (Gilman and Brazeau, 1953):

$$pH = constant + \frac{kidney}{lungs}$$

Calculations of acid-base balance

The Henderson-Hasselbalch equation is important because if any two of the variables (pH, $[HCO_3^-]$ or Pco_2) are known, the third can be calculated. Furthermore, theoretically it allows calculation of what could happen if one of the three variables were changed. For example, if CO_2 is added to the blood, pH and/or $[HCO_3^-]$ must change in a clearly defined way. Measurement or calculation of the three variables allows an accurate assessment of the acid-base balance of the blood. Since normal arterial blood has a pH of 7.40 and pK = 6.10, and

$$pH = pK + \log \frac{[HCO_3^-]}{[CO_2]}$$

$$7.4 - 6.1 = \log \frac{[HCO_3^-]}{[CO_2]} = \log \frac{20}{1}$$

Thus, knowing pK and measuring pH, the $[HCO_3^-]:[CO_2]$ ratio can be calculated. Application of the Henderson-Hasselbalch equation is essential in assessing patients with acid-base abnormalities and these are discussed in the companion volume (Cameron and Bateman, 1983, Chapter 8).

Plasma phosphate buffers

In this system, the acidic ($H_2PO_4^-$) and basic ($NaHPO_4^-$) forms of phosphoric acid are the weak acid and its salt respectively. The system is particularly important in regulating H^+ excretion by the kidney. At pH 7.40, the urine contains four parts of basic for every one part of acidic phosphate. If more acid is excreted and the pH of the urine is reduced to 5.8, the ratio of acidic to basic phosphates becomes 10:1.

In the plasma, phosphate buffers are present but are not very important because the plasma concentrations of free phosphate radicals are small. The pK of the phosphate buffer system is 6.8 (Fig. 6.8), not too far from the blood pH of 7.40. Inside cells, where the pH is probably closer to 7.00, phosphate may be a more important buffer than in plasma or interstitial fluid (Cameron and Bateman, 1983, Chapter 8).

Learning objectives

You should now be able to:

1. define oxygen capacity, saturation and content of blood;
2. describe the structure of haemoglobin;
3. draw and understand the relationships between oxyhaemoglobin saturation, O_2 content and O_2 tension of blood;
4. give the qualitative effects of changes in pH, P_{CO_2}, temperature and 2,3-DPG on the HbO_2-dissociation curve;
5. explain the significance of the differences between adult and fetal haemoglobin;
6. explain the characteristic differences between haemogobin, myoglobin and methaemoglobin;
7. understand what happens in carbon monoxide poisoning;
8. describe the forms in which CO_2 exists in blood and the quantities transported in these forms;
9. draw the relationship between CO_2 content and P_{CO_2} in oxygenated and deoxygenated blood;
10. state the location of carbonic anhydrase and give an account of its function;
11. give an account of the chloride shift;
12. understand what is meant by a buffer and outline the major buffers in blood;
13. understand the pH notation and be able to apply it to the carbonic acid-bicarbonate system (the Henderson-Hasselbalch equation);
14. explain how oxygenation of haemoglobin and its buffering capacity are linked.

7

VENTILATION/PERFUSION RELATIONSHIPS

In ideal lungs, inspiration would supply each of the millions of alveoli with equal amounts of air of uniform composition. Perfusion would distribute to each alveolus an equal amount of mixed venous blood. In the real lung, neither is so. Both ventilation and perfusion increase from apex to base of the lungs due to the effect of gravity. The effect on perfusion is larger because the specific gravity of blood (about 1.0) is greater than that of air-containing lung (about 0.25) (Fig. 7.1). The degree of matching of these two variables is usually expressed as the ratio of ventilation to perfusion ($\dot{V}_A : \dot{Q}$). This ratio determines gas exchange in a region of the lung and normally varies from 0.5 (lung base) to 3.0 (lung apex) (Fig. 7.1).

The majority of this change takes place in the top 25 per cent of the lungs. In the bottom 75 per cent, the lungs do quite a good job at matching ventilation and perfusion. An estimate of how much $\dot{V}_A : \dot{Q}$ inequality interferes with gas exchange in the normal lungs can be made by constructing a mathematical model

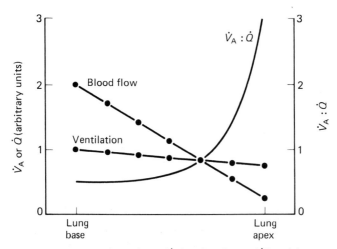

Fig. 7.1 Distribution of ventilation ($\dot{V}_A$) and perfusion ($\dot{Q}$) and the ratio of the two in the upright lung. Both $\dot{V}_A$ and $\dot{Q}$ increase from apex to base, but the $\dot{V}_A : \dot{Q}$ ratio decreases.

of 'ideal' lungs in which ventilation and perfusion are perfectly matched. The model only exchanges 2–3 per cent more O_2 and CO_2 than 'normal' lungs. In diseased lungs, $\dot{V}_A : \dot{Q}$ inequality causes much greater inefficiency.

It should be noted that the *average* $\dot{V}_A : \dot{Q}$ ratio for normal lungs of a resting adult is alveolar ventilation ($\dot{V}_A$) divided by cardiac output ($\dot{Q}$). From the normal values already given, this will be about 4 litre/min divided by 5 litre/min, or 0.8.

The oxygen-carbon dioxide relationship

The $\dot{V}_A : \dot{Q}$ ratios can vary from infinity (dead space, no perfusion) to zero (where blood is shunted through the lungs without coming in contact with the alveolar air). Thus there is a wide range of compositions of alveolar gas and, assuming rapid equilibrium, of capillary blood. A region which is perfused but not ventilated has gas tensions close to those of mixed venous blood, and a region ventilated but not perfused has gas tensions of moist inspired air.

If transfer of O_2 and CO_2 in the lungs were based on a simple mixture effect of blood-borne and ventilation-borne gases, it would be easy to calculate the composition of gas in any alveolus in the same way as we could calculate the composition of the contents of a beaker of saline (i.e. blood) to which various known amounts of water (i.e. alveolar gas) were added (Fig. 7.2).

A very small amount of water added to the beaker of saline leads to a mixture with a composition close to the saline, i.e. the gas tensions will be close to those of venous blood (point v̄ in Fig. 7.2). If a large amount of water is added, or if the amount of saline in the beaker is small, the mixture will have a composition close to that of water; i.e. the capillary gas tensions approach those of the inspired gas (point I in Fig. 7.2). Saline represents the composition of mixed venous blood in non-ventilated regions and water represents the ventilation in regions which are not perfused. The line joining v̄ (non-ventilated) and I (non-perfused) represents

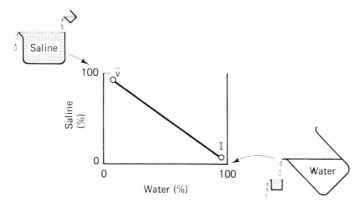

Fig. 7.2 An analogy of under- and overventilated regions of the lung in which the exchange of gases is simplified as the displacement of saline by water.

Saline represents mixed venous blood (v̄) and pure water represents alveolar air (I). Point v̄ represents the composition of blood in poorly ventilated regions of the lung, not enough water being added to wash the salt away. Point I represents regions with ventilation in excess. All the salt is washed away and the composition of I approaches pure water.

different mixtures, or the gas tensions, in lung regions whose $\dot{V}_A:\dot{Q}$s lie between these two extremes. Because the exchange of O_2 and CO_2 in the lung is not a simple displacement of one by the other, the line joining v̄ and I is in fact curved, largely due to the sigmoid shape of the HbO_2 dissociation curve. Chapter 6 describes this in detail.

If a part of the lung is overventilated or underperfused, it blows off extra CO_2 from the blood but it does not absorb extra O_2 because the blood is already 'fully saturated' with O_2 and cannot be more-than-fully saturated. The respiratory gas exchange ratio (R, the ratio of CO_2 output to O_2 uptake, or the respiratory quotient, RQ) is therefore high. Normally the ratio *for the whole lungs* is about 0.8, and varies from 0.7 to 1.0 depending on the food being metabolized (see Chapter 4). Values of R in regions of the lungs with high $\dot{V}_A:\dot{Q}$s can be as high as 2.0. Conversely, if a part of the lungs is underventilated or overperfused, it excretes less CO_2 but still takes up quite a lot of O_2 because of the steepness of the HbO_2-dissociation curve. Values of R in regions of the lungs with low $\dot{V}_A:\dot{Q}$s can be as low as 0.5.

Arterial blood gas measurements

In patients, whether or not regional lung function is investigated, arterial blood gas tensions are often measured as an overall estimate of how well the lungs are doing their job. Regions of impaired function can be better compensated for in terms of CO_2 than O_2 because of the different shapes of their dissociation curves (Fig. 7.3).

Consider what happens if some parts of the lungs are underventilated (low $\dot{V}_A:\dot{Q}$) and others overventilated (high $\dot{V}_A:\dot{Q}$), as often happens in lung disease.

In the case of CO_2, the lung region with a reduced $\dot{V}_A:\dot{Q}$ supplies blood to the pulmonary veins with a high PCO_2 and CO_2 content, while a region with an increased $\dot{V}_A:\dot{Q}$ supplies blood with a low PCO_2 and CO_2 content (Fig. 7.3a). Thus for CO_2, high and low $\dot{V}_A:\dot{Q}$ ratios scattered throughout the lung tend to be self-compensating, the mixture of the blood leaving them being 'normal' in PCO_2 and CO_2 content. *The same is not true for O_2*. A lung region with decreased $\dot{V}_A:\dot{Q}$ supplies blood low in both PO_2 and O_2 content; however, a region with increased $\dot{V}_A:\dot{Q}$ provides a high blood PO_2, but the O_2 content does not increase since the blood is normally full saturated and does not take up more O_2 when PO_2 exceeds 13 kPa (100 mmHg) (Fig. 7.4b). Mixed blood from lung regions with high and low $\dot{V}_A:\dot{Q}$ ratios averages the O_2 *contents*, but this will correspond to a lower-than-average O_2 *tension* because of the shape of the HbO_2-dissociation curve (Fig. 7.4b).

If arterial blood gas tensions are measured, $\dot{V}_A:\dot{Q}$ inequalities in the lungs may cause a low PaO_2, but $PaCO_2$ may be normal. Indeed, $PaCO_2$ may be even lower than normal, if the arterial hypoxia stimulates breathing. If both PaO_2 and $PaCO_2$ in a patient are low, this is very suggestive of excessive $\dot{V}_A:\dot{Q}$ inequalities throughout the lungs.

Arterial PCO_2 is used to define the level of total alveolar ventilation, whether or not there are $\dot{V}_A:\dot{Q}$ inequalities in the lungs, i.e. hyperventilation is defined as a

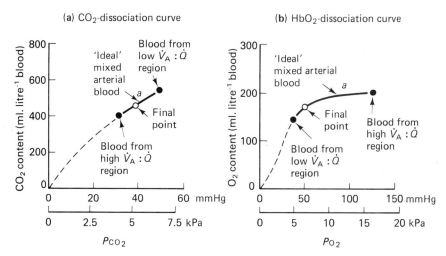

Fig. 7.3 (a) How the near-linear shape of the CO_2-dissociation curve allows for compensation for regional inequalities in $\dot{V}_A : \dot{Q}$ ratios. Areas with high ratios will give off excess CO_2, but this will be balanced by retention of CO_2 in regions with low $\dot{V}_A : \dot{Q}$ ratios. (a) shows the values for CO_2 for 'ideal' lungs with uniform $\dot{V}_A : \dot{Q}$ ratio. The final value for CO_2 in mixed blood from regions with high and low $\dot{V}_A : \dot{Q}$ is close to 'ideal'.

(b) The same mechanism does not apply to O_2, because of the plateau of the HbO_2–dissociation curve. The final value for mixed blood is far below that for 'ideal' lungs.

decrease in Pa_{CO_2} below normal values. Arterial Po_2 values cannot be used in the same way since, if there are $\dot{V}_A : \dot{Q}$ inequalities, the Pa_{O_2} will be low even if total alveolar ventilation is normal.

Nitrogen

Nitrogen dissolved in the blood is not metabolized and so there is no net flux into or out of the body. For the same reason, P_{N_2} is the same in all body fluids. Because the respiratory exchange ratio (R) is generally less than 1, more O_2 is removed than CO_2 is added to alveolar air. Since total alveolar pressure is normally around atmospheric, the decrease in the sum of the partial pressures of O_2 and CO_2 results in a small increase in P_{N_2}. This effect is greatest in regions of the lungs with low $\dot{V}_A : \dot{Q}$ and low R. An increase in P_{N_2} in body fluids such as urine has been suggested as a method of detecting the presence of lung areas with low $\dot{V}_A : \dot{Q}$.

A salutary tale

A student surreptitiously eating peanuts in the library is surprised by the approach of the librarian. He inhales a nut which completely blocks his *right main bronchus*. Leaping about in an attempt to expel the offending fruit, our hero merely succeeds in dislodging a large clot which has formed in a leg vein due to hours of immobility at his studies. If this clot obstructs his *right pulmonary artery*, all will probably be well; although his right lung will be functionally non-existent, his left lung will be normal. if the clot lodges in the *left pulmonary artery*, the consequences of this extreme case of ventilation/perfusion mismatch will be grave. Despite the fact that his *total* lung ventilation and *total* lung perfusion may be adjusted to restore them to normal values, both lungs will be functionally useless, but each for a different reason: one will have no ventilation and one will have no perfusion.

This story may help you understand the importance of matching ventilation and perfusion, and the dangers of an infelicitous lifestyle.

Learning objectives

By now you should be able to:

1. understand the significance of ventilation:perfusion ratio ($\dot{V}_A : \dot{Q}$) and the reasons for its variation;
2. explain how an unusual $\dot{V}_A : \dot{Q}$ ratio will affect the composition of alveolar gas;
3. explain how an unusual $\dot{V}_A : \dot{Q}$ ratio will affect the composition of pulmonary capillary blood;
4. assess how much information about $\dot{V}_A : \dot{Q}$ ratios can be derived from arterial blood gas measurements.

8

CHEMICAL CONTROL OF BREATHING

This chapter is closely related to the next on nervous control of breathing. It could be said that all control of breathing is neural because the afferent elements that sense changes in the external and internal environments which need controlling, and the motor outputs from the brain that bring about this control, are all nervous tissue. However it is convenient to divide control of breathing into chemical and neural components.

The 'responsibilities' of these components have different timings. Neural control operates very rapidly from instant to instant, so that it can change the size and duration of a single breath. Chemical control is generally slower to respond and effects the minute-by-minute ventilation of the lungs. Thus, in general, chemical control determines minute ventilation and neural control determines the pattern by which the ventilation is made up.

All the systems of the body are concerned with homeostasis (maintenance of the internal environment). Respiration is particularly concerned with homeostasis in terms of O_2 – providing energy for other systems – and CO_2 – closely related to $[H^+]$ (see Chapter 6). Because they sense the chemical composition of the arterial blood, those tissues that act as sensors in the chemical control of breathing are called *chemoreceptors*. They can be described in terms of site and sensitivity. Those situated within the central nervous system are called central chemoreceptors, and those outside the central nervous system are peripheral chemoreceptors. The latter are primarily sensitive to lack of O_2 and the former to excess of CO_2.

Lack of oxygen

The general term for lack of O_2 is *hypoxia*, and the specific term for lack of O_2 in the arterial blood is *hypoxaemia*. The absolute absence of O_2 is *anoxia*.

Sensors of hypoxia

These are the peripheral chemoreceptors, the carotid bodies and aortic bodies, which are small (5.0 mm diameter) nodules of glomus tissue (Fig. 8.1). Although

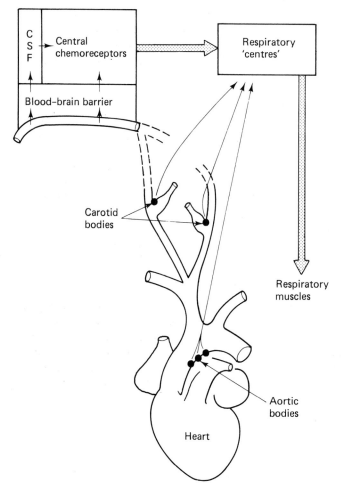

Fig. 8.1 The central and peripheral chemoreceptors. The carotid bodies are bilaterally situated, one at each carotid bifurcation, and their afferent fibres are in the glossopharyngeal nerves. The aortic bodies have afferent fibres in both vagus nerves. The central chemoreceptors are on the ventrolateral surface of the medulla and are supplied with cerebrospinal fluid and with materials that penetrate the blood-brain barrier.

the carotid bodies are close to regions of the arterial system that regulate blood pressure, they are not baroreceptors. The carotid bodies receive their arterial blood supply from the internal or external carotid arteries and send their information to the brain in the glossopharyngeal nerves. The aortic bodies are scattered around the aortic arch and send their information to the brain in the vagus nerves.

The embryology of the peripheral chemoreceptors is physiologically interesting. As a mammalian embryo develops, its structure passes through stages resembling more primitive species (ontogony recapitulates phylogony). During the fish-like phase those structures which are going to become the O_2-sensitive chemoreceptors of the adult are represented by the gill arches of the fish-like embryonic form, and it is the gills of fish which are sensitive to O_2 lack in their surrounding water. So our peripheral chemoreceptors may represent a residue of the mechanism by which our fishy ancestors detected low O_2 in their watery environment.

Anatomically the peripheral chemoreceptors contain Type I and Type II cells and nerve fibres (Fig. 8.2). The Type I cells are thought to be the actual site stimulated by hypoxia to release a transmitter which stimulates sensory nerve endings. Type II cells resemble supporting or glial cells in nervous tissue and they probably do not have functional connections with nerve fibres. There is much controversy as to the mechanism of peripheral chemoreceptor response to hypoxia, what if any is the transmitter between Type I cells and nerve fibres, and what is the physiological role of the sympathetic and parasympathetic nerve supply to the chemoreceptors. These motor nerves appear, experimentally at least, to modify their sensitivity by changing blood flow through them.

Chemoreceptor response to hypoxia

The peripheral chemoreceptors are unusual in being stimulated by hypoxia. Most other parts of the body are depressed by hypoxia. The ventilatory response of a subject on being given increasingly hypoxic gas to breathe (and therefore having his arterial Po_2 reduced) is shown in Fig. 8.3. Inspired Po_2 must be reduced considerably (to about half that of normal room air) before breathing is significantly stimulated. Subsequently a very low partial pressure of O_2 depresses breathing.

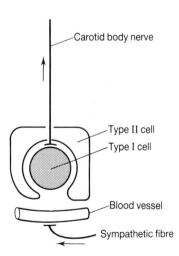

Carotid body nerve

Type II cell

Type I cell

Blood vessel

Sympathetic fibre

Fig. 8.2 Diagram of cell types and nerve fibres in a carotid body. Note the carotid body receives both afferent and efferent fibres.

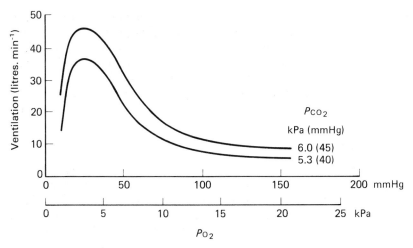

Fig. 8.3 Ventilatory responses to O_2 at different values of Pco_2. Note that very low alveolar Po_2 suppresses breathing.

Stimuli to peripheral chemoreceptors

Although the actual stimulus to and the intrinsic mechanisms of the peripheral chemoreceptors are not clear, the essential physiological observations in relation to breathing are as follows.

1. The chemoreceptors have an exceptionally large blood flow (weight for weight, 40 times that of the brain) so venous blood leaving them is almost fully saturated with O_2. Thus they 'taste' the Po_2 of carotid artery blood, and are not stimulated by anaemia (when blood O_2 content is low but O_2 tension is normal); however severe circulatory depression (stagnant hypoxia) does activate the chemoreceptors.
2. The chemoreceptors have a remarkably high metabolic rate and so use up a large part of the O_2 provided to them by their high blood flow.
3. Low PaO_2 stimulates peripheral chemoreceptors and increases breathing. Moderate decreases in PaO_2 cause only small increases in breathing, and only severe hypoxia has a large effect.
4. Increases in PaO_2 above normal (13 kPa, 100 mm Hg) produced by inhaling O_2-rich mixtures only slightly depress breathing by inhibiting the chemoreceptors.
5. Increases in arterial $[H^+]$ do not affect central chemoreceptors directly but increase breathing by stimulating peripheral chemoreceptors.
6. Peripheral chemoreceptors also respond to increases in $PaCO_2$ but are far (10 or more times) less sensitive than the central chemoreceptors in this respect.
7. The activity of the peripheral chemoreceptors can be modified by sympathetic motor activity, which reduces blood flow through them and increases their sensitivity to hypoxia, and by parasympathetic activity which decreases their sensitivity.

All these facts support the view that the actual stimulus to the peripheral chemoreceptors is a build-up of metabolites which takes place when the rate of supply of O_2 to the chemoreceptors is not sufficient for its metabolic needs. This dependence on O_2 supply, which depends in turn on blood flow, explains why peripheral chemoreceptors are activated in two situations which pose a serious threat to life: hypotension due to haemorrhage, and hypoventilation causing asphyxia.

Hypoxia and breathing

The oxyhaemoglobin dissociation curve (page 63) shows that even if alveolar Po_2 falls to approximately 8 kPa (62 mm Hg) haemoglobin will still be 90 per cent saturated. Similarly, Po_2 can rise to infinity and haemoglobin can only be 100 per cent saturated. Thus, because of the shape of the oxyhaemoglobin dissociation curve, ventilation can halve or double without there being significant changes in the amount of O_2 carried by the blood. A mechanism which relied on O_2 saturation to control breathing under normal circumstances would therefore lack sensitivity. Nevertheless the peripheral chemoreceptors are very important because they are the only mechanism in the body by which low O_2 tension can stimulate breathing.

Not only is the hypoxic mechanism of the peripheral chemoreceptors relatively insensitive, but it also tends to be opposed by the CO_2 and $[H^+]$ regulating mechanisms. Thus, when breathing is stimulated by hypoxia, CO_2 is washed out from the blood, arterial $[H^+]$ falls, and the drive to breathe from these two sources is reduced, in part neutralizing the effects of hypoxia (the 'hypocapnic brake' – see Fig. 8.4). If this braking effect is prevented, ventilation will increase by up to 10 times more as a result of hypoxia, which indicates just how powerful a stimulus pure hypoxia can be.

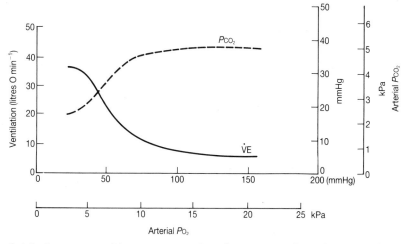

Fig. 8.4 Braking action of hypocapnia resulting from increased ventilation (produced by hypoxia) on that ventilation. As hypoxia increases (curves move to left), Pco_2 decreases and, although ventilation ($\dot{V}_E$) increases the size of the change is reduced by the hypocapnia.

Chronic hypoxia

The response of the body to low PaO_2, such as is encountered when one goes to high altitude and stays there for several days, is different from the pattern of acute changes we have discussed so far. These chronic changes, which largely involve washing out CO_2 from the blood and the subsequent adaptation of central receptors to the new level of CO_2, are dealt with in Chapter 10. In certain lung diseases the reduced ability of the lungs to transfer O_2 to the blood also produces hypoxaemia and the response of the body to this condition is in many respects similar to the response to high altitude.

Other actions of peripheral chemoreceptors

As well as increasing breathing, stimulation of peripheral chemoreceptors:

1. constricts peripheral blood vessels (except those in the skin);
2. increases heart rate;
3. increases activity of the adrenal glands.

These three activities combine to increase blood pressure.

Although the peripheral chemoreceptors require large changes in inhaled PO_2 before they stimulate breathing, they are important because:

1. they are the only place in the adult body where hypoxia can stimulate respiration;
2. they respond to CO_2 excess as well as O_2 lack and so can maintain the response to CO_2 excess when central receptors are depressed; and
3. they respond to CO_2 excess more rapidly (in seconds) than do the central chemoreceptors (in minutes).

Excess of carbon dioxide

The major chemical factor regulating ventilation is CO_2. High levels of CO_2 are known as *hypercapnia* and low levels as *hypocapnia*. There is normally very little CO_2 in the surrounding air (0.03 per cent). Any increase in inhaled CO_2 stimulates breathing in a near linear manner (Fig. 8.5) until either the CO_2 load causes an intolerable sensation of suffocation or the blood PCO_2 reaches such a high value that it begins to depress breathing. Very high concentrations of CO_2 are an effective general anaesthetic.

Site and sensitivity of central chemoreceptors

Unlike the response to hypoxia (Fig. 8.3), small increases in inhaled CO_2 will produce an increase in breathing (Fig. 8.5). This stimulation begins fairly quickly in response to a step-wise change in arterial PCO_2 (within 20 s), but equilibrium takes about 5 min.

This timing can be understood since the areas sensitive to CO_2 are the peripheral chemoreceptors of the carotid and aortic bodies and the central chemoreceptors situated just below the surface (500 μm) of the ventrolateral

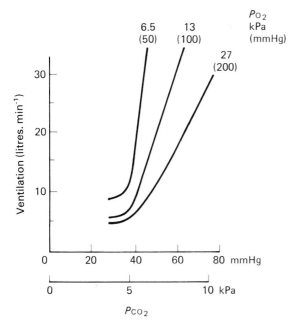

Fig. 8.5 Ventilatory responses to CO$_2$ at different values of Po_2. Note the inflection of the curves (dogleg) at about 4kPa (30 mmHg); not all authors give this dogleg for high Po_2.

regions of the medulla oblongata (Fig. 8.6a). The peripheral chemoreceptors respond quickly to changes in Pco_2, and the central receptors which are responsible for about 80 per cent of the total response react more slowly.

The blood–brain barrier

No precise structures have been identified in the regions indicated in Fig. 8.6a as being sensitive to CO$_2$, but it is presumed that nerve endings in these regions are stimulated by changes in interstitial fluid (ISF). The composition of ISF bears a complicated relationship with that of cerebrospinal fluid (CSF), and both are influenced by the blood–brain barrier. This barrier greatly restricts and controls the movement of ions (but not O$_2$ and CO$_2$) between CSF and the plasma from which it is made at the choroid plexus (Fig. 8.6b).

Increased CO$_2$ in arterial blood rapidly diffuses across the blood–brain barrier into the ISF and the CSF. Here it displaces the reaction

$$CO_2 + H_2O = H_2CO_3 = H^+ + HCO_3^-$$

to the right, with the production of H$^+$ which is probably the specific stimulus to the chemoreceptors.

Although investigation of these central chemoreceptors has been carried out using artificial and modified CSF, it is probably the ISF inside the tissue just below the lateral and ventral surfaces of the medulla which is important. CSF composition influences this, as does the tendency of the blood–brain barrier to

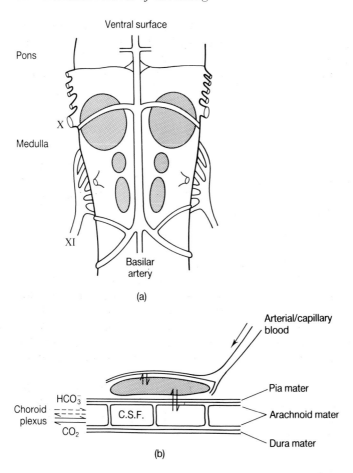

Fig. 8.6 (a) location of central chemosensitive areas (stippled) on ventral surface of the medulla. (b) Postulated relationship between such areas (stippled) and blood and cerebrospinal fluid. Solid arrows indicate passive CO_2 diffusion; interrupted arrows indicate active bicarbonate transport.

keep the composition of CSF as near to normal as possible. These compensatory changes are of particular importance in chronic (24 hours or more) changes in blood CO_2 such as are produced at altitude and during chronic lung disease.

Small decreases in blood CO_2 due, for example, to voluntary hyperventilation, usually have little depressant action on breathing (except in subjects who know a little about respiratory physiology and think that they should stop breathing). The $P_{CO_2}/\dot{V}_E$ curve that defines the subject's sensitivity to CO_2 flattens along what is colloquially called the dogleg (Fig. 8.4). Presumably during hyperventilation other afferent inputs keep breathing going even in the absence of stimulation from the central chemoreceptors.

The sensitivity of breathing to an increase in P_{CO_2} varies from person to person, but on average an increase in P_{aCO_2} of 0.3 kPa (2.5 mm Hg) will double minute ventilation if other factors are constant. H^+ cannot pass directly through the blood–brain barrier, so increases in blood $[H^+]$ do not affect the central chemoreceptors provided arterial P_{CO_2} is constant. The medullary chemoreceptors are not stimulated by reductions in blood P_{O_2}; in fact severe hypoxia depresses breathing in adults by a direct action on the brainstem respiratory complex.

Asphyxia

Isolated changes in either arterial P_{O_2}, P_{CO_2} or $[H^+]$ are rare unless imposed by physiologists. The three are usually changed at the same time, and the breathing response is the sum of their interactions. These interactions were expressed by Gray as long ago as 1945 in the following formula:

$$VR = 0.22[H^+] + 0.262\ P_{CO_2} - 18 + 105/10^{0.038}\ P_{O_2}$$

where VR is the ratio of alveolar ventilation to its rest value.

The importance of this formula is not in its numerical accuracy, but in its illustration that no single chemical factor controls respiration. The usual stimulus to breathing is asphyxia, and the synergistic interaction between reduced P_{O_2} and increased P_{CO_2} is illustrated in Fig. 8.4 where the slopes of the $P_{CO_2}/\dot{V}_E$ curves are seen to steepen with progressive hypoxia, producing a greater response to the combination of stimuli than might be expected from their simple sum.

The factors controlling ventilation have already been seen to 'moderate' the effects of each other. Thus the braking effect of the washing out of CO_2 from the blood of a subject exposed to the hypoxia of altitude moderates a hyperventilation which could lead to alkalosis and tetany.

Learning objectives

By now you should be able to:

1. explain how control of breathing is part of the regulation of the internal environment;
2. understand the different roles of chemical and neural controls of breathing;
3. describe the locations and adequate stimuli for the chemoreceptors;
4. state the effects of changes in Pa_{O_2}, Pa_{CO_2} and $[H^+]$ on breathing;
5. state the relative potency of the above stimuli;
6. discuss the interaction of chemical stimuli on breathing.

9

NERVOUS CONTROL OF BREATHING

Pattern of breathing

Breathing is unusual among the automatic systems of the body. We have seen in the previous chapter that, left undisturbed, it goes about its day-to-day business of controlling O_2, CO_2 and $[H^+]$ in the body. However, unlike the heart of kidneys, the respiratory system can be subjugated to voluntary tasks such as talking, or can be used to assist in other tasks such as lifting weights or playing the trumpet. The nervous control of breathing also enables the body to choose a particular pattern of breathing to achieve a minute ventilation appropriate for its metabolic needs at that time.

Minute ventilation is governed by chemical control to ensure homeostasis of O_2, CO_2 and $[H^+]$. Minute ventilation ($\dot{V}_E$) is given by the equation

$$\dot{V}_E = V_T \times f$$

where V_T and f are the tidal volume of each breath and the frequency of breathing. From this equation it follows that a particular minute ventilation could be made up of an infinite combination of volumes and frequencies, ranging from high frequencies combined with small tidal volumes to low frequencies combined with large tidal volumes. However each individual 'chooses' one particular combination of frequency and volume for a particular minute ventilation.

The pattern of breathing chosen relates to the amount of work required to produce a particular minute ventilation. This work is directly related to the force exerted by the respiratory muscles. Factors that determine the amount of such work have been dealt with in Chapter 3, and it seems that the optimum pattern of breathing is chosen to minimize the total amount of work done and/or the force produced by the respiratory muscles. This optimal pattern of breathing is controlled by a rhythm generator in the brainstem, modulated by various afferent inputs. Neural activity leaves the central nervous system via the phrenic and intercostal nerves, among others, to bring about breathing by contractions of the respiratory muscles, mainly the diaphragm and intercostals.

Origin of respiratory rhythm

In the central nervous system there is a central rhythm generator which produces a basic, 'rough and ready' pattern of breathing. This pattern is modified and refined by other regions of the brain and by afferent information from receptors in the lungs and chest to produce a pattern which is efficient and responsive to changing conditions.

The origin of respiratory rhythm is in that part of the brainstem which joins the spinal cord to the mid-brain and cerebellum, and which is shown in Fig. 9.1 and in more detail in Fig. 9.4. The region consists of the medulla and the pons, which joins the medulla to the rest of the brain. If the medulla is carefully isolated from all the structures above it, which can therefore no longer influence respiration (see Fig. 9.3, transection II), breathing is remarkably normal in pattern. Breathing is only abolished by transection between the medulla and the spinal cord. (There is, however, some evidence of rhythm generators in the spinal cord.) Thus the major rhythm generator seems to be situated in the medulla and is influenced by higher regions of the brain and by reflex activity from other parts of the body.

How the actual rhythm (inspiration followed by expiration, followed by inspiration, etc.) is generated is still something of a mystery. There could be a reciprocal interaction between the two groups of neurons that produce inspiration and expiration (Fig. 9.2a), an old but persistent idea with little evidence to support it. A more recent concept is that the inspiratory neuron pool not only

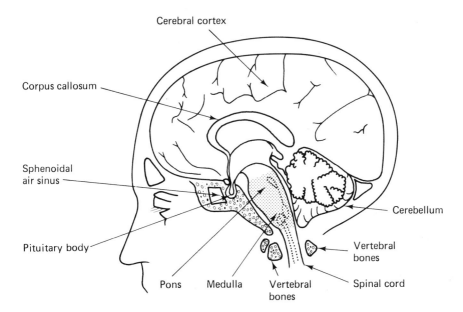

Fig. 9.1 A section of the brain and skull showing the structures involved in breathing. The brainstem, the site of origin of respiratory rhythm, is shaded. The main respiratory areas and pathways in the brainstem are dotted.

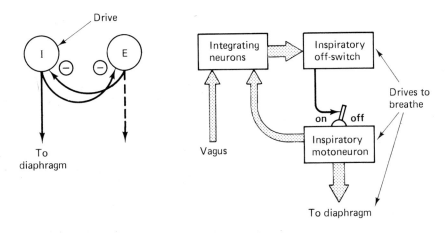

(a) Oscillator model   (b) Off-switch model

Fig. 9.2 (a) The oscillator model of control of respiratory rhythm. Inspiratory (I) and expiratory(E) groups have neurons that rhythmically wax and wane as their inhibitory influence on each other gains and loses dominance. (b) The off-switch model. Inspiratory motoneuron activity is terminated by 'off-switch' neurons. This off-switch is activated by the summation of vagal drive from pulmonary stretch receptors and feedback from the inspiratory motoneurons themselves. Other inputs can either change the activity of the off-switch, modify intrinsic level of activity of the inspiratory motoneurons or bypass the rhythm generator to control directly the respiratory muscles.

contracts the inspiratory muscles, but also activates a negative-feedback loop in the medulla that triggers an 'off-switch' which limits inspiration (Fig. 9.2b). Whether or not this is so, the facts about the physiology of the rhythm generator are as follows.

1. All the inspiratory neurons are linked and all the expiratory neurons are similarly linked by self-exciting connections which synchronize their activities.
2. Inspiratory and expiratory neuron groups are each self-inhibiting, at least in normal breathing, to limit the duration of their activities;
3. If the expiratory neuron pool is active in eupnoea (quiet breathing), its motor action down the spinal cord does not reach a level which activates the main expiratory muscles – those of the abdominal wall – since expiration in eupnoea is passive.

The respiratory neuron groups

Experiments over the last 100 years or more which involved transecting the brainstem in the region of the pons with or without cutting both vagus nerves resulted in abnormal patterns of breathing (Fig. 9.3). These results led to the erroneous idea of anatomical 'centres' in the pons which, with the reflexes from the peripheral nervous system, modified the activity of the medullary rhythm generator into an efficient pattern appropriate to the conditions in which the animal found itself. The term 'respiratory centre' is incorrect in that it implies a

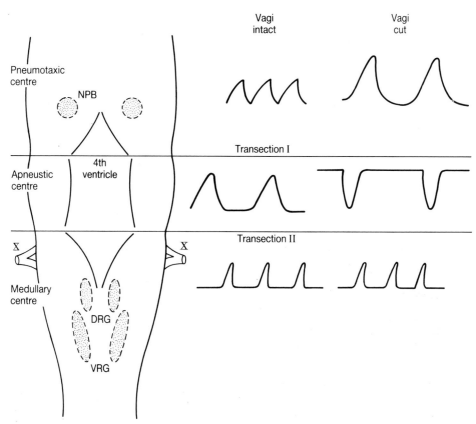

Fig. 9.3 Brainstem structures involved in breathing. NPB, Nucleus parabrachialis medialis (pneumotaxic centre); DRG, Dorsal respiratory group (nucleus of the solitary tract); VRG, Ventral respiratory group (nucleus ambiguus and nucleus retroambigualis). Changes in breathing pattern due to removal of the influence of the upper pons or vagi. Removal of either alone slows and deepens breathing while removal of both causes apneusis.

discrete anatomical entity while the functional reality is more in the nature of a diffuse network of neurons which are active together.

If the upper pons is disconnected from the medulla (Transection I, Fig. 9.3) the influence of the so-called pneumotaxic centre is removed. The neurons that make up this 'centre' are probably situated in or close to the nucleus para-brachialis medialis. This centre was discovered by the observation that, when the upper pons is destroyed, breathing becomes slower and deeper (Fig. 9.3). It is believed that every time the inspiratory neuron group of the medulla discharges, it not only contracts the diaphragm but also sends impulses up to the pneumotaxic centre which, after a delay, sends impulses back to the inspiratory cells to cut short their burst of activity by negative feedback. The pneumotaxic centre would therefore have a rate-controlling, volume-limiting mechanism, and we can speculate that it has evolved as a relay to mediate the rapid shallow breathing that can be initiated from even higher parts of the brain in conditions such as thermal or emotional panting.

The time and volume limiting effects of the pneumotaxic centre on breathing are seen properly only if the vagi are cut because either the pneumotaxic centre or the vagi can carry out this role.

The apneustic centre is another 'centre' postulated to exist in the lower pons. If the pneumotaxic centre is removed by Transection I (Fig. 9.3), breathing is slower and deeper if the vagi are intact. If the vagi are also cut, the absence of the two mechanisms (both of which limit inspiration) leads to apneusis – long and powerful inspiratory efforts interspersed with brief expirations. This was once explained by the existence of an 'apneustic centre' in the lower pons. However it is more likely that apneusis is a functional derangement than that an anatomical apneustic centre exists.

The dorsal and ventral respiratory groups

The abnormal patterns of breathing described above, seen in experimental animals with brainstem lesions, can also be seen in patients with damage in this region – clocklike unmodulated rhythms, slow deep patterns of breathing and apneusis. These observations suggest that our brainstems are organized in a way similar to those of other animals. From other observations, two functionally distinct groups of neurons in the medulla have been identified, mainly by recording action potentials and selective staining of neurons (see Fig. 9.4).

The *dorsal respiratory group* (DRG) of neurons is in the region of the nucleus tractus solitarius. From this region the DRG receives and integrates information about breathing from chemoreceptors and mechanoreceptors. It has been suggested that the cells of the DRG and nearby nerves have a spontaneous rhythm and may act as a pacemaker from which the basic rhythm of breathing originates.

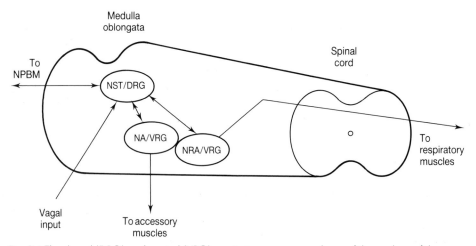

Fig. 9.4 The dorsal (DRG) and ventral (VRG) respiratory groups made up of the nucleus of the solitary tract (NST); the nucleus ambiguus (NA) and the nucleus retroambigualis (NRA). These structures are shown on one side of the medulla only together with their connections to the respiratory muscles and the nucleus parabrachialis medialis (NPBM).

The *ventral respiratory group* (VRG), unlike the DRG, consists of both inspiratory and expiratory upper motorneurons. Inspiratory activity in the DRG excites inspiratory cells and inhibits expiratory cells in the VRG. The VRG is concentrated rostrally in the nucleus ambiguus and caudally in the nucleus retroambigualis. The rostral part innervates accessory muscles of respiration (such as those in the larynx) on the same side. The caudal part innervates the contralateral diaphragm, the contralateral expiratory intercostal and abdominal muscles, and the ipsilateral and contralateral inspiratory intercostal muscles.

The two pontine centres already mentioned, the pneumotaxic centre and the more speculative apneustic centre, probably exert their influence via the VRG.

Voluntary control of breathing

In anaesthetized animals, areas of the brain above the pons usually have little action on breathing. The hypothalamus, cerebral cortex and cerebellum can be removed without greatly changing or interfering with breathing, or its chemical or neural control. However, in unanaesthetized man, not only do higher centres involuntarily affect breathing in conditions such as hyperthermia, emotion and possibly exercise, but also we can control our respiratory muscles voluntarily. This voluntary control is always bilateral, for example we cannot contract half our diaphragm. Its origin is unknown but may be in the motor cortex. What is certain is that the voluntary pathways bypass the pneumotaxic centre and the respiratory rhythm generator in the brainstem and descend in the pyramidal tracts (Fig. 9.5). A patient whose voluntary pathways have been destroyed, by a stroke for example, may still breathe normally and respond to reflex and chemical stimuli, but cannot voluntarily control his or her own breathing. Such a patient will cough if the larynx is stimulated but not if he or she tries to initiate it deliberately. The opposite dissociation is sometimes seen with severe brain damage; if the pyramidal tracts are intact the patient can breathe deliberately, but natural automatic breathing is lost and he or she has to be artificially ventilated when sleeping. This rare condition was mentioned in Chapter 1 (page 9).

This separation of the pathways for voluntary and automatic breathing persists in the spinal cord. The voluntary pathways from the cerebral cortex pass down the lateral areas of the spinal cord, whereas the automatic pathways from the respiratory regions of the brainstem are more anterior, near the outlets of the ventral roots (Fig. 9.5).

The muscles of breathing

The expiratory motoneurons of the spinal cord are inhibited during inspiration, and the inspiratory motoneurons are inhibited during expiration. This reciprocal inhibition prevents opposing inspiratory and expiratory muscle groups contracting together. Unlike opposing skeletal muscle systems, this inhibition is not mediated via muscle-spindle reflexes but originates in the dorsal and ventral respiratory groups.

It would be difficult for the muscle spindle system of reciprocal inhibition to

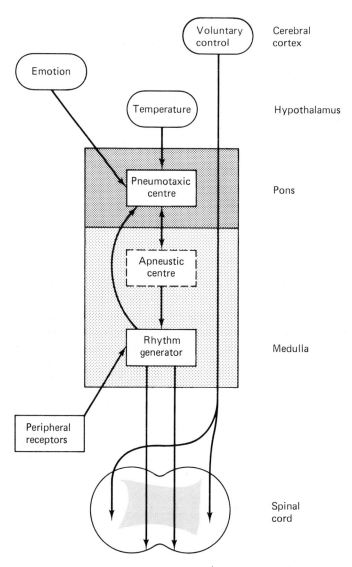

Fig. 9.5 Diagram of the main nervous structures controlling breathing. The brainstem respiratory complex is shaded. At the bottom, the main pathways in the spinal cord are indicated.

work for the diaphragm because it has very few muscle spindles. The diaphragm is controlled almost entirely by direct motor fibres (alpha-motoneurons) from the cervical region. These alpha-motoneurons are unusual in that they lack feedback to Renshaw cells which, for other motoneurons, cut short after-discharge of activity. The other respiratory muscles, the intercostals and abdominals, behave in general more like most other skeletal muscles and both have respiratory and postural functions. The external intercostals cause inspiration and the internal intercostals cause expiration. These intercostal muscles have an abundance of muscle spindles. Their contraction is caused by a combination of direct activation of extrafusal muscle fibres plus indirect activation via stimulation of the intrafusal fibres of muscle spindles which produces reflex contraction.

Both groups of intercostal muscles are active in quiet breathing, but the abdominal muscles only have a respiratory role in forced expiration, as in coughing and exercise. It is remarkable how the muscles of the chest wall and abdomen can play a major and varying role in posture and locomotion, and at the same time both breathing and the refined modifications of airflow in speech can be precisely and effectively superimposed on this varying activity. We can breathe and talk whilst undertaking almost any form of exercise and in almost any posture.

Reflex modification of breathing

Lung reflexes

One of the most important inputs controlling pattern of breathing travels to the brainstem in the Xth cranial (vagus) nerves. The vagus nerves carry afferent information from other parts of the body, but that from the lungs is of paramount importance in control of breathing. These lung reflexes come from three types of receptors. The slowly adapting pulmonary stretch receptors and the rapidly adapting receptors, which send their information in large and small-diameter myelinated fibres respectively, and C-fibre receptors which send their information in small-diameter nonmyelinated fibres.

Slowly adapting pulmonary stretch receptors
When a constant stimulus is applied to a receptor, the rate of discharge of that receptor decreases even though the stimulus does not change (Fig. 9.6).

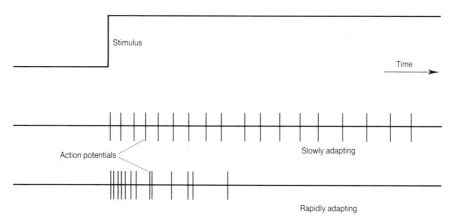

Fig. 9.6 The response of slowly and rapidly adapting receptors to the application of a constant stimulus.

Receptors can be classified as slowly adapting, if their rate of discharge decreases slowly (Fig. 9.6a), or rapidly adapting if it decreases quickly, despite the stimulus remaining the same (Fig. 9.6b). Receptors of both type are found in the lungs and send impulses up the vagus nerves to modify the pattern of breathing.

Slowly adapting receptors in the lungs respond to stretch of the airways and signal to the brain the volume of the lungs at any moment. During inspiration this activity increases and it has been postulated to operate an 'off-switch' (see Fig. 9.2) which terminates inspiration in terms of duration and volume. This off-switch effect is most clearly seen in the Breuer-Hering inflation reflex in which the lungs of an anaesthetized animal are inflated and it ceases to make inspiratory efforts for some time. Cutting the vagus nerves abolishes this reflex. During the first part of expiration, while the lungs are deflating, the stretch receptors are still active but their activity wanes as the lungs empty.

The slowly adapting receptors are situated in the smooth muscle of the trachea and bronchi and so are influenced by factors that affect bronchial tone. Many have a tonic discharge throughout the expiratory pause of normal breathing. In addition to inhibiting inspiration and lengthening expiration, they also cause a reflex bronchodilation and accelerate the heart.

Since rhythmical breathing exists after bilateral vagotomy, the activity of lung stretch receptors is not essential for rhythm but only modifies the pattern of breathing (without having a large effect on total minute volume at rest). The advantage of this modulating influence may be that it adjusts the pattern of breathing to be most economical in terms of work or force of breathing (see Chapter 3). In animals the pattern of breathing becomes more expensive in terms of work when the vagus nerves are cut since slow deep breathing requires more energy than normal breathing. The mechanical work of breathing depends on the compliance of the lungs and the airways resistance. The activity of pulmonary stretch receptors is affected by changes in lung compliance and resistance, usually in a way that reflexly alters pattern of breathing to minimize work. For example, a reduction in lung compliance sensitizes stretch receptors (since stiffer lungs cause a greater pull on the large airways where the receptors lie), which in turn produces more shallow and rapid breathing which is more efficient in this condition.

The importance of slowly adapting receptors in the control of quiet breathing in unanaesthetized man has been disputed, since large inflations (over 1 litre) are required to inhibit respiration. However the receptors are present in the lungs and they may play a different role. The Breuer-Hering reflex is present in man during sleep and activity from slowly adapting receptors has been recorded in the vagus nerves of humans.

During hyperpnoea, more rapid lung inflation causes slowly adapting receptors to reach a level of activity that operates the respiratory off-switch earlier than normal. Inspiratory duration is shortened and breathing frequency increases. In man this probably only occurs with large tidal volumes. The fact that the receptors also reflexly dilate the bronchi and accelerate the heart may be an advantage in reducing airways resistance and increasing cardiac output in exercise.

Although stretch receptors are primarily mechanosensitive, they are inhibited by an increase in P_{CO_2} (hypercapnia). This may play a part in shortening the expiratory phase when breathing is stimulated by CO_2.

Rapidly adapting receptors (irritant receptors)
The discharge of these receptors, as their name implies, rapidly adapts to a constant mechanical stimulus (Fig. 9.6b). Thus in breathing, where the stimulus is constantly changing, their discharge is highly erratic and difficult to quantify. Perhaps this is the reason why they have received, until recently, much less attention from investigators than the more regularly firing, slowly adapting stretch receptors. Their alternative name, irritant receptors, arises from the fact that they can be stimulated by such irritating substances as ammonia gas and cigarette smoke and during pneumothorax (air in the pleural space). These are clearly not the physiological stimuli the receptor would encounter under normal conditions and therefore 'rapidly adapting receptor' is a more suitable name. They have also been called 'deflation receptors' since they are stimulated by deflation and contribute to the Breuer-Hering deflation reflex. Their true physiological stimulus is probably rate of change of lung volume, which is related to air-flow into or out of the lungs.

Their rapidly adapting pattern of discharge is similar to that of receptors in the larynx and trachea that cause cough and, like these receptors, they probably consist of free nerve-endings lying close to the surface of the epithelium of the airways and concentrated particularly at divisions of the airways. Unlike cough receptors in the trachea and larynx, the rapidly adapting receptors in the lungs provoke rapid shallow breathing when stimulated, mainly by shortening the duration of expiration.

They also cause the deep augmented breaths which mammals take periodically (every 5–20 min in resting man). These breaths reverse the slow collapse of the lungs which takes place during quiet breathing. The ability of rapidly adapting receptors to provoke augmented breaths appears to be 'gated' at some point because, when an augmented breath has occurred, it is impossible to provoke another for some time. This phenomenon explains how it is possible for rapidly adapting receptors to produce the apparently diametrically opposite effects of deep slow (augmented) breaths and rapid shallow breathing that are seen when they are stimulated.

By their property of terminating expiration, rapidly adapting receptors may have a role in initiating inspiration both in normal breathing and in the first deep gasps of a newborn infant.

Apart from these physiological roles, rapidly adapting receptors are strongly activated by inhalation of irritant gases and particles and by a number of lung diseases. They may be responsible for the changes in breathing pattern seen with many lung diseases and perhaps the sensation of dyspnoea (breathlessness) that occurs under these conditions. As well as increasing minute ventilation, rapidly adapting receptors cause the reflex bronchial and laryngeal constrictions and airway mucus secretion often seen in lung disease.

C-fibre receptors (J-receptors)
A third group of lung receptors that send information to the brainstem in the

vagus nerves have thin nonmyelinated C-fibres. In the lungs the receptors are situated close to the pulmonary capillaries, and hence the alternative name of J-(juxtapulmonary capillary) receptors. A similar group of receptors is in the bronchial wall and are called bronchial C-fibre receptors. The receptors are stimulated by increases in interstitial fluid (oedema) and by substances such as histamine, bradykinin and prostaglandins which are released during lung damage. The vagal reflex response to C-fibre receptor stimulation is apnoea or rapid shallow breathing, fall in heart rate and blood pressure, laryngeal constriction, airway mucus secretion and relaxation of skeletal muscles by inhibition of spinal motoneurons, and a general depression of somatic and visceral activity which would be appropriate in serious lung damage. A clear role for pulmonary C-fibre receptors in normal breathing has yet to be demonstrated.

Non-pulmonary reflexes

The pattern of breathing changes when one stubs one's toe, and the hilarity of such an event changes the pattern of breathing in observers. Thus pain and emotion can alter the pattern of breathing via nervous pathways from higher regions in the central nervous system to the respiratory areas of the brainstem. Impulses from other parts of the body can also affect respiration.

Reflexes from the respiratory muscles
Just like other skeletal muscles, but unlike the diaphragm, the respiratory muscles of the thoracic cage have an abundance of muscle spindles which provide a feedback mechanism operating at a spinal level. This mechanism seems to provide a load-detecting reflex so that an extra load in the form of decreased compliance or increased resistance applied to the respiratory system is rapidly compensated for by increased drive to the extrafusal muscles; these develop additional tension and so contribute to proper maintenance of ventilation.

Reflexes from the nose and pharynx
Stimulation of nerve endings within the nose can provoke a sneeze. This consists of a deep inspiration followed by a closure of the glottis which allows pressure to build up so that the subsequent expiratory movement is sufficiently violent to remove the stimulating material. It is interesting that a sneeze, unlike a cough, is difficult to suppress voluntarily or to mimic. In many subjects a bright light will provoke a sneeze, but the mechanism is unknown.

Irritation of the nasopharynx can produce a sniff or aspiration reflex. This has the form of a sharp intake of air and presumably serves to clear material from the back of the nose.

Reflexes during swallowing
During swallowing respiration is inhibited in whatever phase of the respiratory cycle swallowing is initiated. This reflex has obvious protective value in preventing inhalation of food.

The cough reflex
Coughs can be elicited from the upper airways, and particularly the larynx, by stimulating superficial rapidly adapting receptors. Unlike the rapidly adapting receptors deeper in the lungs, whose stimulation in general produces rapid shallow breathing, cough receptors produce a rather similar reflex to the sneeze. There is a deep inspiration followed by a closure of the glottis to provide a high-pressure blast of air to expel the irritating substances through the mouth.

Reflexes from visceral and somatic regions
Passive movements of a limb reflexly increase breathing in both anaesthetized animals and conscious man. This may contribute to the increase in ventilation seen in exercise.

Cold water applied to the skin promptly and dramatically increases minute ventilation by a mechanism other than the distress produced by this unpleasant experience.

Visceral pain generally produces opposite effects on breathing to those caused by somatic pain. Thus distension of the intestine, gallbladder or bile duct inhibits breathing, and traction on some of the viscera can cause apnoea.

Learning objectives

By now you should be able to:

1. describe the sites and functions of the regions of the brain necessary for a normal respiratory pattern;
2. state why 'respiratory centre' is not a precise term;
3. give an account of at least six afferent neural influences (including four reflexes) on the rhythm generator;
4. discuss the termination of inspiration;
5. outline the motor innervation of the respiratory muscles;
6. describe how the voluntary control of the respiratory muscles differs from the automatic;
7. explain how expiration may be active or passive.

10

SPECIAL RESPIRATORY CONDITIONS

Birth

At the birth of a baby the cardiovascular–pulmonary changes are the most dramatic of its lifetime. While a fetus, a mammal makes shallow respiratory movements at regular intervals and occasionally gives large gasps, probably exercising its respiratory muscles for the moment after birth when its umbilical cord is cut and it must breathe or die.

What initiates breathing? Certainly the multiple and strange sensory stimuli which bombarded the neonate produce arousal. The tissues are using O_2 and producing CO_2, so very soon peripheral and central chemoreceptors are strongly stimulated. In a full-term baby all the sensory receptors are properly connected by nervous pathways to the 'respiratory centres', and the latter are connected to the respiratory muscles. In the very premature infant this is not so. Since fetal lungs contain liquid, the first breath requires an unusual effort. The first inspiration must pull fluid 36 times more viscous and 1000 times more dense than air through the small airways. When the baby's head emerges first from the birth canal, the thorax is squeezed so that it is emptied of some of its liquid; the attendant physician may also clear the mouth and nose of liquid. Nevertheless, a transpulmonary pressure of as much as 8 kPa (60 mmHg) may be needed to overcome all the resisting factors of the first breath, although such a high pressure could not be maintained for long.

The first expirations are also important. If all the air from inspiration was expelled, the lungs would revert to their collapsed fetal state, with cohesion of the walls of the alveolar ducts and bronchioles. The second inspiration would require the same tremendous effort as the first and breathing would soon exhaust the infant. This does happen in infants with respiratory distress syndrome, which is frequently associated with prematurity. The Type II cells of these infants' lungs have not yet made enough surfactant to ensure alveolar stability (see Chapter 2). Normally, a fairly stable functional residual capacity is built up within a few minutes of birth. Presumably, once the lungs contain gas, even the forced expirations of crying do not expel all of it because some is retained by the dynamic airway closure described in Chapter 3. Pulmonary circulation increases rapidly when air first enters the lungs, and this aids the speedy absorption of amniotic fluid.

Breathing is maintained in the infant because inhibitory influences that were present in the uterus have been removed and because arousing stimuli are present. A positive feedback reflex from the lungs stimulates large inspiratory efforts similar in mechanism to augmented breaths in the adult (see Chapter 9), and may be important in the period immediately after birth.

High altitude

The common clinical condition of hypoxia is somewhat analogous to ascent to high altitude by a normal individual. The fall in barometric pressure on ascent causes a reduction in atmospheric partial pressure of O_2. Arterial Po_2 is therefore also decreased, causing stimulation of peripheral chemoreceptors and increase in ventilation. This hyperventilation washes out CO_2 from the blood and cerebrospinal fluid and both liquids become more alkaline. This respiratory alkalosis reduces the drive to breathe and masks the respiratory stimulation due to the hypoxia. After one to two days, the blood–brain active transport system returns the $[H^+]$ of the CSF towards normal. This restored drive together with that from the reduced arterial Po_2 progressively increases ventilation over this period. During the first one to two weeks at altitude the kidney excretes extra HCO_3^- and restores blood $[H^+]$ towards normal; this blood change excites the peripheral chemoreceptors even more, increasing ventilation even further. Figure 10.1 summarizes some of the breathing changes during acclimatization to altitude.

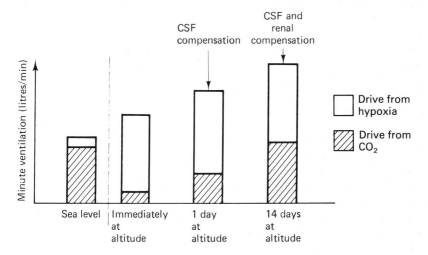

Fig. 10.1 The way breathing acclimatizes to high altitude during a few days. Immediately on reaching high altitude, low Po_2 causes hyperventilation which washes out CO_2 (and therefore H+) from the blood and CSF. The drive to breathe due to CO_2 is restored in two overlapping stages, corresponding to compensations in the CSF and kidneys. The hypoxic drive remains constant.

A number of other adaptations to altitude occur, including an increase in the number of red blood cells, a shift in the HbO_2-dissociation curve to the right, and an increase in pulmonary arterial pressure due to pulmonary vasoconstriction.

Space flight

The ultimate in high altitudes must be space flight. In this the astronaut must take his own atmosphere. This could be either air at normal atmospheric pressure (the Soviet system), or pure O_2 at low total pressure (the American system). Pure O_2 at one atmosphere is toxic over long periods, so the gas mixture and pressure have to be adjusted to give a normal alveolar Po_2 of about 13 kPa (100 mmHg). Since the alveoli also contain CO_2 at a pressure of 5.5 kPa (40 mmHg) and water vapour at 6.1 kPa (47 mmHg), pure O_2 at a pressure of 25 kPa (200 mmHg) is about right. The choice of the system depends largely on engineering considerations.

To escape from the Earth's gravitational field, a space ship must reach a velocity of 11600 m. s^{-1}. While it is being accelerated to this speed, the body is subjected to high gravitational forces which increase the weight of the tissues and displace those relatively free to move. We have seen in Chapters 4, 5 and 7 that gravity is a major cause of non-uniform distribution of ventilation and perfusion in the lung. If a man were accelerated only gently in a 'headwards' direction, i.e. standing up in his rocket ship, blood would not reach the top of his lungs so that alveoli ventilated there would become dead space; the blood flow at the bottom of the lungs would become an arteriovenous shunt since alveoli there would be collapsed by the gravitational force and would have no ventilation. For this reason astronauts are positioned at right angles to the direction of movement of the rocket or capsule during acceleration and deceleration. An alternative theoretical arrangement would be a return to the womb; astronauts would be surrounded by and 'breathe' O_2 dissolved in liquid of the same density as their bodies. This would render their lungs immune to the effects of acceleration. This has already been tested, but only in anaesthetized animals.

Temperature

Many animals use their respiratory systems to regulate body temperature. In a hot environment they increase their minute volume (hyperpnoea), and water evaporating from their airways carries with it its latent heat of vaporization. To minimize hyperventilation and loss of CO_2, the panting pattern of breathing is rapid and shallow, so that alveolar ventilation increases far less than does total ventilation. To lessen the work of this increased breathing, animals often resort to mouth breathing and probably also dilate their larynx to reduce total airways resistance. Goats can increase their rate of breathing from about 40 to 270 breaths per minute as a result of a rise in body temperature of 1°C. This pattern of breathing is not so mechanically undesirable as it might appear, since the breathing frequency is close to the resonant frequency of the respiratory system. This minimizes the increase in mechanical work of breathing required. Priority is given to the control of temperature over the regulation of blood gas composition and, in spite of the shallowness of the breathing, Pa_{CO_2} falls precipitously. Many mammals are covered in fur and have few sweat glands, so they cannot, like man, rely on efficient evaporation of sweat from their skin to control body temperature.

Humans, and some other species that can sweat efficiently, do not pant during hyperthermia, although there may be a tendency to rapid/shallow breathing with hyperventilation. The unpleasant effects of spending too long relaxing in a very hot bath may, in part, be due to hypocapnia and decreased arterial $[H^+]$, which are the price paid for a small gain in evaporative cooling by increased ventilation. Since hyperthermia in resting humans produces hyperventilation, it has been suggested that an increase in body temperature during exercise may be involved in control of breathing in this condition. However, changing the core temperature of people carrying out different levels of work does not greatly change their ventilation until core temperature exceeds 39°C, which is an appreciable heat stress.

Water as well as heat is lost via the respiratory system. Dehydration in a hot environment is well known. It may seem paradoxical, but a great deal of water is also lost in this way in very cold climates. Cold air contains very little water vapour even when fully humidified. When it is inspired it is warmed to body temperature and saturated with water in the lungs. This water is partly but not completely deposited in the cooler parts of the nose on expiration and the rest condenses in the atmosphere, as the clouds of breath on a winter's day will testify. For this reason, polar explorers run the risk of suffering from dehydration, surrounded by a sea of fresh water, albeit frozen. Some animals, such as the camel, can lessen the loss of water vapour during a cold desert night by breathing out cold dehumidified air from the nose, the water presumably being trapped in hygroscopic material in the nasal air passages.

Breathing in sleep

Simple observation of sleeping subjects suggests that two fairly distinct respiratory patterns may occur. Sometimes breathing seems regular and appears normal, as in a relaxed awake person. At other times breathing is irregular, often with occasional very deep breaths and long apnoeic pauses. Snoring may be observed with either pattern, but is more usual with the second.

Neurological investigations confirm that sleep can be generally divided into two categories, usually identified by changes in the activity of the brain, displayed as an electroencephalogram (EEG). The slow waxing and waning of EEG activity in the quietly sleeping subject or animal is disrupted when sleep passes into the more active stage, and the two categories can be identified by physical signs as follows.

Quiet sleep

Wakefulness merges into quiet sleep through a series of stages categorizing the depth of sleep. There is a progressive reduction in muscle tone. Breathing is slower and deeper than when awake, and there may be a small increase in arterial

$P\text{CO}_2$. Vagal feedback reflexes such as the Breuer-Hering reflex may be stronger in animals and become apparent in humans. The sensitivity of the subject to inhaled CO_2 or to hypoxia is probably unchanged. In general, the subject acts like a lightly anaesthetized person, except that most forms of anaesthesia depress the respiratory control system in the brainstem.

Active (REM) sleep

This deeper level of sleep is marked by jerky movements of the body, rapid eye movements (REM), and loss of muscle reflexes. Breathing is irregular, with on average an increase in frequency and decrease in tidal volume. In man arterial $P\text{CO}_2$ is unchanged or slightly decreased; in spite of this the subject shows diminished responses to inhaled CO_2 and hypoxia. Lung reflexes seem to be inhibited. The cough reflex is also depressed and stimulation of the larynx may now cause apnoea; an important defensive mechanism is thereby lost. Thus there is a general depression of the breathing response to mechanical and chemical stimuli.

Snoring and obstructive sleep apnoea

The pharynx is a region of the upper airways particularly lacking in support from bone or cartilage. As it is also extrathoracic it is not supported by negative intrapleural pressure as are the smaller, intrathoracic airways. In both forms of sleep – quiet and active – there is relaxation of the muscles of the larynx, pharynx and mouth. For these reasons, and particularly when the air-pressure inside the pharynx becomes excessively negative during inspiration (due to nasal airways obstruction for example), the pharynx tends to collapse, obstructing its airway. Extra effort is required to force air through this obstruction, and the pharynx rapidly 'flaps' open and closed and the palate vibrates, producing the characteristic sound of snoring. This can occur in both the inspiratory and expiratory phases of breathing but is usually more marked in inspiration. It is estimated that at least a quarter of the adult population habitually snore.

Snoring is a very emphatic signal that the pharyngeal obstruction is being overcome, albeit as the result of some considerable effort. A more sinister situation arises when, due to the strength of the obstruction, the subject cannot draw breath through the obstructed pharynx. Obstructive sleep apnoea then arises. This cessation of breathing is usually only resolved by the subject waking up, which may happen hundreds of times per night, but for periods too brief for the subject to remember. As the obstruction usually occurs during REM sleep, the subject is deprived of this essential part of sleep which can result in personality changes and daytime sleepiness and lead to accidents while driving or using machinery.

Breathing under water

Diving is similar to life *in utero* in that the subject is surrounded by liquid, but differs in that the lungs and several other body spaces are filled with gas which, unlike tissues and tissue fluid, is compressible. The gas is the origin of many of the problems encountered. These problems confront both scuba (self-contained underwater breathing apparatus) divers and the more old-fashioned 'hard-hat' divers whose head and body are surrounded by an air-containing helmet and suit connected to an air compressor on the surface. In either case the diver must be supplied with air at almost the same pressure as the water surrounding him – the inspiratory muscles are not strong enough to overcome the pressure of more than a few feet of water. The efforts of early divers who attempted to work while connected to the surface by a simple tube held in the mouth were frustrated by this effect. Therefore, as one dives deeper the lungs must be filled with air at greater absolute pressure.

Two gas laws are relevant to some of the problems encountered by divers. Boyle's Law tells us that the volume of a fixed mass of gas varies inversely with its pressure. Gas in the gut, the lungs, the middle ear and sinuses is compressed on diving and expands on return to the surface. If the diver is supplied with compressed air, its pressure is kept equal to that of his surroundings. On descent, which is relatively slow, this air enters the lungs, middle ear and sinuses, and there is no serious problem. However, if from depth he quickly ascends to the surface, there can be serious problems. The gas in his body will expand: if, as is normal, this gas is freely connected to his surroundings via open mouth and nose, no difference in pressure develops. The gas expands and escapes from the body, and no damage is done. All divers are taught very early in their careers that they must breathe out when making a rapid ascent. Pressure increases by about 1 atmosphere for each 10 m descended beneath water surface. The effect on the lungs of a diver surfacing from only 40 m if he held his breath would be catastrophic, since his lung volume would expand fivefold and his chest would explode. Gas trapped in ears and sinuses is not always freely connected to the outside and its expansion can be painful.

The fact that the respired gas is compressed causes further problems. Since its density and viscosity are increased the work of breathing is greater. In addition, the voice becomes far lower in pitch since the resonant properties of the sinuses and air passages depend on the physical properties of the respired gas.

Henry's Law tells us the amount of a gas which dissolves in blood and body fluids is proportional to the gas's partial pressure. The deeper a person dives and the greater the pressure of gas supplied to him, then the amounts of gas dissolved in his body are larger. During descent there is no problem, but on return to the surface gas may come out of solution and form bubbles in the muscles and joints, causing severe pain (the bends). Bubbles in the peripheral and central nervous systems can cause sensory disturbances and convulsions. The answer to this problem is to bring the diver slowly to the surface, which allows the dissolved gas time to diffuse out of the body via the bloodstream and lungs and to be expired before it can form bubbles. The problem is largely one of N_2. Any bubbles of CO_2 and of O_2 would be rapidly excreted in expired air or used in metabolism. These problems of decompression could be eliminated by giving the diver 100 per cent O_2 to breathe, but O_2 at pressures above 1 atmosphere is toxic if breathed for long. The usual solution is for the diver to breathe a mixture of O_2 and a gas such as He which is less soluble than N_2. With such a mixture, the amount and rate at which the inert gas dissolves are reduced but not eliminated.

Exercise

Gas exchange in exercise

It is a function of the lungs to provide appropriate amounts of oxygen and to remove carbon dioxide at all levels of metabolism.

In severe exercise, O_2 uptake (and CO_2 output) can increase twentyfold (from 0.25 litres . min^{-1} at rest to 5 litres . min^{-1}) and alveolar ventilation shows a corresponding increase. Three factors limit this increase in O_2 uptake.

The first is the maximal minute ventilation that can be maintained, and therefore the amount of O_2 that can be made available in the lungs. Voluntary maximal breathing capacity (MBC) is about 150 litres . min^{-1} in laboratory conditions, but in exercise a ventilation of 120 litres . min^{-1} is about the limit which an average young adult can achieve without rapid exhaustion, and corresponds to a fifteenfold increase in minute and alveolar ventilation.

The second limit to O_2 uptake is the amount of O_2 that can be removed from alveolar gas. Normally the 21 per cent O_2 in inspired air is reduced to about 14 per cent in alveolar air, which means that fully saturated arterial blood leaves the lungs; to extract a much higher percentage of O_2 from the alveolar air would be self-defeating because the blood leaving the lungs would be less saturated and would carry O_2 to the tissues at a lower tension (see Chapter 6). Venous blood would be even more desaturated than usual.

The third limit to O_2 uptake is the pulmonary blood flow or cardiac output. This is normally about 5 litres . min^{-1} at rest, and can increase to about 25 litres . min^{-1} in severe exercise. Although it might at first seem that the uptake of O_2 can therefore only increase fivefold, it must be remembered that during exercise the tissues are extracting a far greater amount of O_2 from the blood. At rest, mixed venous blood is about 75 per cent saturated, but in severe exercise its O_2 content may be only a third of this (25 per cent saturated). Thus, although, with the given figures, the *carriage* of O_2 from the lungs only increases fivefold, the greater *extraction* of O_2 by the tissues causes a three times greater desaturation of blood returning to the lungs, so that the *uptake* and *usage* of O_2 are fifteen times larger, which corresponds to the increase in ventilation mentioned above.

In moderate exercise, initially the increase in O_2 uptake may exceed that of CO_2 output, since the tissue stores of CO_2 (mainly as HCO_3^-) are large and take time to be mobilized. Therefore, the respiratory exchange ratio (R) may be lower than normal at the start of moderate exercise (Fig. 10.2).

If the O_2 supply to muscle is inadequate, anaerobic metabolism takes place, i.e. energy-releasing processes which do not require O_2 are brought into play. At this *anaerobic threshold*, lactic acid is formed from glycogen and released into the bloodstream causing a non-respiratory acidosis (see Chapter 6). After exercise, about four-fifths of the lactic acid is converted back into muscle glycogen, and the other one-fifth is metabolized to provide the energy for this conversion. During the release of lactic acid in exercise, CO_2 output in the lungs increases above that due to CO_2 formation in aerobic metabolism, because of the action of lactic acid on blood bicarbonate (Fig. 10.2). As a result, the respiratory exchange ratio (R) may exceed 1. After exercise, when the lactic acid is removed

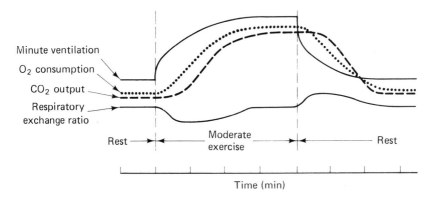

Minute ventilation
O₂ consumption
CO₂ output
Respiratory exchange ratio

Rest — Moderate exercise — Rest

Time (min)

Fig. 10.2 Changes in minute ventilation, O_2 consumption, CO_2 output and respiratory exchange ratio (R) during a period of uniform moderate exercise, without anaerobic metabolism. Note that the beginning of exercise the increase in O_2 uptake exceeds that of CO_2 output, with a fall in R.

from the blood, CO_2 is retained, and R may be less than 0.7. This retention of CO_2 after exercise is sometimes called repayment of the O_2-debt of anaerobic metabolism in exercise; the amount of CO_2 retention after exercise is proportional to the amount of lactic acid released in the exercise, which in turn is proportional to the extent to which the muscles lacked O_2 and had to rely on anaerobic metabolism.

Control of breathing in exercise

It is not clear what stimuli provoke the increase of ventilation during exercise. Two facts must be borne in mind while searching for such stimuli:

1. in moderate steady exercise lung ventilation is proportional to O_2 uptake, CO_2 output and to metabolic rate (Fig. 10.3);
2. there is an abrupt increase in breathing at the beginning of exercise and an abrupt decrease at the end of it (see Fig. 10.2).

Carbon dioxide
Exercise produces extra CO_2, so this seems a strong candidate for the stimulus of breathing in exercise. However, all chemoreceptors so far discovered are supplied with arterial blood, and there is little change in arterial P_{CO_2} even when exercise has produced a fifteenfold increase in ventilation. Such a ventilatory response would require an arterial P_{CO_2} as high as 10 kPa (75 mmHg) in the absence of exercise.

Another possibility is that exercise increases the sensitivity of the respiratory centre to inputs from peripheral or central chemoreceptors. This is unlikely because the slope of the CO_2-response curve is the same when exercising and at rest.

It is clear that, although the mechanism that increases ventilation in exercise is powerful, it does not overcome the homeostatic mechanism that controls arterial

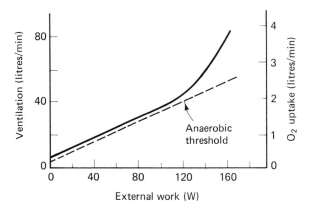

Fig. 10.3 Relationship between ventilation (solid line) and O_2 uptake (interrupted line) during increasing levels of exercise. At low levels, the two variables increase proportionally. But above a certain level of work, at the anaerobic threshold, ventilation increases disproportionately.

Note that the resting metabolic rate requires some O_2 uptake and ventilation even when no external work is being done.

The actual value of the anaerobic threshold depends on the fitness and training of the subject and the type of external work.

Pco_2. However, blood CO_2 could still be an important stimulus. If CO_2 is artificially added to *venous blood* returning to the heart, ventilation increases considerably before a Pco_2 increase can be detected in the arterial blood. The experiment suggests that there may be receptors in the venous side of the circulation which detect the increase in venous return of CO_2 in exercise and stimulate breathing. This attractive concept has often been advocated, but receptors sensing CO_2 in the venous system have not yet been identified.

Another possibility is based on the fact that during exercise the fluctuations in arterial Pco_2 due to the respiratory cycle are much greater than at rest, although

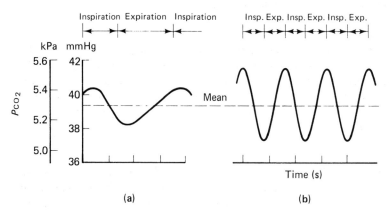

Fig. 10.4 Changes in alveolar Pco_2 (a) at rest and (b) during exercise. The oscillations in Pco_2 are greater in exercise but the means are identical.

the average P_{CO_2} is unchanged (Fig. 10.4). Neurophysiological studies show that chemoreceptors are sensitive to the rate of change of the chemical stimulus as well as to the mean strength of the stimulus, and it has been suggested that it is the oscillatory pattern of discharge of the chemoreceptors that provides the respiratory stimulus in exercise.

The relative stability of arterial P_{CO_2} even in rather severe exercise needs to be stressed. This is physiologically desirable because of the ease with which CO_2 enters the brain and changes $[H^+]$ there. Whatever mechanisms increase ventilation in exercise, they do so in association with a CO_2-control system of great sensitivity, so that any 'errors' in this control system and consequent changes in Pa_{CO_2} are small or indetectable. In a theoretically perfect system there would be no error, i.e. no change in the variable (P_{CO_2}) which is being controlled.

Hypoxia as a stimulus
The other side of the high P_{CO_2} coin is low P_{O_2}. However, only in severe exercise is there an appreciable decrease in arterial P_{O_2}. Also, as with CO_2, no hypoxia sensors have been found on the venous side of the circulation. It has been suggested that blood flow to the arterial chemoreceptors is sharply decreased during exercise by vascular reflexes so that the chemoreceptors are activated in spite of a normal arterial P_{O_2}. This idea is not supported by the observation that patients who have had their carotid bodies surgically removed increased ventilation on exercise but not during hypoxia. However, the facts remain that O_2 consumption (and therefore aerobic metabolism) is closely correlated to ventilation, and breathing pure O_2 during severe exercise reduces ventilation by 10 per cent.

Hydrogen ion concentration as a stimulus
Since anaerobic metabolism during exercise leads to an increase in blood lactic acid, the resulting acidosis could stimulate breathing via the peripheral chemoreceptors. However, the arterial $[H^+]$ changes seem to be too small to account for most of the ventilatory increase in exercise.

Unknown substances
Failure to detect significant changes in arterial P_{O_2}, P_{CO_2} and $[H^+]$ led to the suggestion that some unknown substance may be active in stimulating respiration. If such a substance exists, it does not work by exciting receptors in veins or in the pulmonary circulation. When blood trapped in an exercising limb by an occluding cuff is released, it does not stimulate breathing until it reaches the systemic arteries.

Increased temperature
Blood from exercising tissues is warmer than normal and this could increase breathing by an action on structures in the brain. Such a mechanism could not explain the immediate hyperpnoea of exercise. However, the gradual decrease to normal ventilation after exercise has the same time course as the change in body temperature, although this could be a coincidence.

Impulses from the motor cortex
It has been suggested that when muscles are activated from the motor cortex of the brain, signals proportional to those going to the muscles are sent simultaneously to the respiratory centres. This would explain the rapid increase and decrease in ventilation at the beginning and end of exercise. However, the slow changes during and after exercise must be due to other factors.

Mechanoreceptors in muscles and joints
Passive movements of a limb stimulate breathing, probably by activation of receptors in and around joints, and this could contribute to the respiratory changes in exercise.

Conditioned responses
There is often an increase in ventilation before exercise begins, provided the subject knows what is about to happen. This is not a deliberate voluntary effect but must depend on conscious anticipation of exercise.

Multiple factor hypothesis
The inability to find a single mechanism to explain the regulation of ventilation in exercise has led to the concept that multiple factors are involved. Many mathematical equations which predict, with greater or lesser success, ventilation under given conditions of exercise have been produced. Perhaps the greatest value of these efforts has been to make it clear that the influence of each factor varies with the type of exercise, its intensity, duration and environmental factors, and that the stimulation of breathing in exercise is unlikely to be due to a single mechanism.

In this section on exercise we have gone to some length to show the uncertainty that exists in our understanding of one of the most important aspects of respiratory control – exercise hyperpnoea. A similar approach could have been made to many of the other aspects of breathing which are presented in a far more dogmatic way. It is regrettably necessary to oversimplify subjects which, at the research level, are controversial and often ill-understood.

Learning objectives

By now you should be able to:

1. outline the respiratory changes that take place at birth;
2. discuss the respiratory difficulties the newborn may meet;
3. outline the short- and long-term respiratory and chemical changes brought about by ascent to high altitude;
4. understand the respiratory problems related to space flight and to diving under water;
5. describe the respiratory changes in hyperthermia, and its effect on water balance;
6. describe the changes of breathing induced by sleep, including snoring;

7. outline ventilation and gas exchange as a function of intensity of work during steady muscular exercise;

8. outline the changes in ventilation and respiratory quotient at onset, during, and at the end of exercise;

9. define and explain the anaerobic threshold and describe what happens when it is exceeded;

10. list the factors which may be important for increasing ventilation during exercise.

FURTHER READING

Chapter 1 Lung structure and function

Cameron, I. and Bateman, N. (1983). *Respiratory Disorders*. Edward Arnold, London.

Comroe, J. H. Jr (1974). *Physiology of Respiration*, 2nd edn. Year Book, Chicago.

Horsfield, K. (1986). Morphometry of the lungs. In *Handbook of Physiology, Section 3, The Respiratory System*. Vol III Mechanics of breathing, Part I, p. 75. Edited by P. T. Macklem and J. Mead. American Physiological Society, Bethesda.

Martin, D. E. and Youtsey, J. W. (1988). *Respiratory Anatomy and Physiology*. C. V. Mosby, St Louis.

Murray, J. F. (1988). *The Normal Lung*, 3rd edn. W. B. Saunders, Philadelphia.

Nagaishi, C. (1973). *Functional Anatomy and Histology of the Lungs*. University Park Press, Baltimore.

Porter, R. and Whelan, J. (eds.) (1980). *Metabolic Activities of the Lung*. Ciba Foundation Symposium 78. Excerpta Medica, Amsterdam.

Satir, P. and Sleigh, M. A. (1990). The physiology of cilia and mucociliary interactions. *Annual Review of Physiology*, **52**, p. 137.

Weibel, E. R. (1983). Is the lung built reasonably? *American Review of Respiratory Disease*, **128**, p. 752.

Weibel, E. R. (1985). Lung cell biology. In *Handbook of Physiology, Section 3, The Respiratory System*. Vol I Circulatory and nonrespiratory functions, p. 47. Edited by A. P. Fishman and A. B. Fisher. American Physiological Society, Bethesda.

West, J. B. (1989). *Respiratory Function: The Essentials*, 4th edn. Blackwell, Oxford.

Chapter 2 Pressure and volume

Bangham, A. D. (1987). Lung surfactant: how it does and does not work. *Lung*, **165**, p. 17.

Bourbon, J. R. and Rientort, M. (1987). Pulmonary surfactant: biochemistry, physiology and pathology. *News in Physiological Sciences*, **2**, p. 129.

Cameron, I. and Bateman, N. (1983). *Respiratory Disorders*. Edward Arnold, London.

Cotes, J. E. (1979). *Lung Function: Assessment and Application in Medicine*, 4th edn. Blackwell, Oxford.

Goerke, J. and Clements, J. A. (1986). Alveolar surface tension and lung surfactant. In *Handbook of Physiology, Section 3, The Respiratory System*. Vol III Mechanics of breathing, Part I, p. 247. Edited by P. T. Macklem and J. Mead. American Physiological Society, Bethesda.

Hills, B. A. (1988). *The Biology of Surfactant*. Cambridge University Press, Cambridge.

Macklem, P. T. (1978). Respiratory mechanics. *Annual Review of Physiology*, **40**, p. 157.

Van Golde, L. M. G., Batenburg, J. J. and Robertson, B. (1988). The pulmonary surfactant system: biochemical aspects and functional significance. *Physiological Reviews*, **68**, p. 374.

West, J. B. (1987). *Pulmonary Physiology: The Essentials*. Blackwell, Oxford.

Chapter 3 The dynamics of lung ventilation

Barnes, P. J. (1986). Neural control of human airways in health and disease. *American Review of Respiratory Disease*, **134**, p. 1289.

Cameron, I. and Bateman, N. (1983). *Respiratory Disorders*. Edward Arnold, London.

Comroe, J. H. Jr (1974). *Physiology of Respiration*, 2nd edn. Year Book, Chicago.

Macklem, P. T. (1978). Respiratory mechanisms. *Annual Review of Physiology*, **40**, p. 157.

Mortola, J. P. (1987). Dynamics of breathing in newborn mammals. *Physiological Reviews*, **67**, p. 244.

Orehek, J. (1981). Neurohumoral control of airway calibre. In *MTP International Review of Physiology*, Vol 23, p. 1. Edited by J. G. Widdicombe. University Park Press, Baltimore.

Rodarte, J. R. and Rehder, K. (1986). Dynamics of respiration. In *Handbook of Physiology, Section 3 The Respiratory System*. Vol III Mechanics of breathing, Part I, p. 131. Edited by P. T. Macklem and J. Mead. American Physiological Society, Bethesda.

Chapter 4 Lung ventilation

Anthonisen, N. R. and Fleetham, J. A. (1987). Ventilation: total, alveolar, and dead space. In *Handbook of Physiology, Section 3, The Respiratory System*. Vol IV Gas exchange, p. 113. Edited by L. E. Farhi and S. M. Tenney. American Physiological Society, Bethesda.

Cameron, I. and Bateman, N. (1983). *Respiratory Disorders*. Edward Arnold, London.

Cerretelli, P. and di Prompero, P. E. (1987). Gas exchange in exercise. In *Handbook of Physiology, Section 3, The Respiratory System*. Vol IV Gas exchange, p. 297. Edited by L. E. Farhi and S. M. Tenney. American Physiological Society, Bethesda.

Comroe, J. H. Jr (1974). *Physiology of Respiration*, 2nd edn. Year Book, Chicago.

Cotes, J. E. (1979). *Lung Function: Assessment and Application in Medicine*, 4th edn. Blackwell, Oxford.

Forster, R. E. and Crandall, E. D. (1976). Pulmonary gas exchange. *Annual Review of Physiology*, **38**, p. 69.

Otis, A. B. (1987). An overview of gas exchange. In *Handbook of Physiology, Section 3, The Respiratory System*. Vol IV Gas exchange, p. 1. Edited by L. E. Farhi and S. M. Tenney. American Physiological Society, Bethesda.

West, J. B. (1987) Pulmonary gas exchange. In *MTP International Review of Physiology*, vol 14, p. 83. Edited by J. G. Widdicombe. University Park Press, Baltimore.

West, J. B. (1990). *Ventilation/Blood Flow and Gas Exchange*, 5th edn. Blackwell, Oxford.

Chapter 5 Pulmonary circulation

Cameron, I. and Bateman, N. (1983). *Respiratory Disorders*. Edward Arnold, London.

Daly, I. De B. and Hebb, C. (1966). *Pulmonary and Bronchial Vascular Systems*. Edward Arnold, London.

Dawson, L. A. (1984). Role of pulmonary vasomotion in physiology of the lung. *Physiological Reviews*, **64**, p. 544.

Fishman, A. P. (1985). Pulmonary circulation. In *Handbook of Physiology, Section 3, The Respiratory System*. Vol I Circulation and nonrespiratory functions, p. 93. Edited by A. P. Fishman and A. B. Fisher. American Physiological Society, Bethesda.

Fishman, A. P. (1988). Normal pulmonary circulation. In *Pulmonary Diseases and Disorders*, Vol 2. McGraw-Hill, New York.

Gil, J. (1980). Organization of microcirculation of the lung. *Annual Review of Physiology*, **42**, p. 177.

West, J. B. (ed.) (1976). *Regional Differences in the Lung*. Academic Press, London.

West, J. B. (1977). Pulmonary gas exchange. In *MTP International Review of Physiology*, Vol 14, p. 83. Edited by J. G. Widdicombe, University Park Press, Baltimore.

West, J. B. (1990). *Ventilation/Blood Flow and Gas Exchange*, 5th edn. Blackwell, Oxford.

Chapter 6 Blood gas transport and pH

Adamson, J. W. and Finch, C. A. (1975). Haemoglobin function, oxygen affinity, and erythroprotein. *Annual Review of Physiology*, **37**, p. 351.

Bartels, H. and Bauman, R. (1977). Respiratory function of haemoglobin. In *MTP International Review of Physiology*, Vol 14, p. 107. Edited by J. G. Widdicombe. University Park Press, Baltimore.

Bauer, C., Gros, G. and Bartels, H. (eds.) (1980). *Biophysics and Physiology of Carbon Dioxide*. Springer-Verlag, New York.

Bauman, R., Bartels, H. and Bauer, C. (1987). Blood oxygen transport. In *Handbook of Physiology, Section 3, The Respiratory System*. Vol IV Gas exchange, p. 147. Edited by L. Farhi and S. M. Tenney. American Physiological Society, Bethesda.

Cameron, I. and Bateman, N. (1983). *Respiratory Disorders*. Edward Arnold, London.

Jones, N. L. (1980). *Blood Gases and Acid-Base Physiology*. Marcel Dekker, New York.

Klocke, R. A. (1987). Carbon dioxide transport. In *Handbook of Physiology, Section 3, The Respiratory System*. Vol IV Gas exchange, p. 173. Edited by L. Farhi and S. M. Tenney. American Physiological Society, Bethesda.

Michel, C. C. (1974). The transport of oxygen and carbon dioxide by the blood. In *MTP International Review of Physiology*, Vol 2, p. 67. Edited by J. G. Widdicombe. University Park Press, Baltimore.

Perutz, M. F. (1990). Mechanisms regulating the reactions of human haemoglobin with oxygen and carbon dioxide. *Annual Review of Physiology*, **52**, p. 1.

Chapter 7 Ventilation/perfusion relationships

Cameron, I. and Bateman, N. (1983). *Respiratory Disorders*. Edward Arnold, London.

Comroe, J. H. Jr (1974). *Physiology of Respiration*, 2nd edn. Year Book, Chicago.

Farhi, L. E. (1966). Ventilation-perfusion relationship and its role in alveolar gas exchange. In *Advances in Respiratory Physiology*, p. 148. Edited by C. A. Caro. Edward Arnold, London.

Farhi, L. E. (1987). Ventilation-perfusion relationships. In *Handbook of Physiology, Section 3, The Respiratory System*. Vol IV Gas exchange, p. 199. Edited by L. E. Farhi and S. M. Tenney. American Physiological Society, Bethesda.

Rahn, H. and Fenn, W. O. (1955). *A Graphical Analysis of the Respiratory Gas Exchange: The O_2–CO_2 Diagram*. American Physiological Society, Washington DC.

Weibel, R. E. (1984). *The Pathway for Oxygen: Structure and Function in the Mammalian Respiratory System*. Harvard University Press, Cambridge, MA.

West, J. B. (1976). *Regional Differences in the Lung*. Academic Press, London.

West, J. B. (1990). *Ventilation/Blood Flow and Gas Exchange*, 5th edn. Blackwell, Oxford.

Chapter 8 Chemical control of breathing

Acker, H. (1989). PO_2 chemoreception in arterial chemoreceptors. *Annual Review of Physiology*, **51**, p. 835.

Bruce, E. N. and Cherniack, N. S. (1987). Central chemoreceptors. *Journal of Applied Physiology*, **62**, 389.

Cummin, R. C. and Saunders, K. B. (1987). The ventilatory response to inhaled CO_2. In *The Control of Breathing in Man*, p. 45. Edited by B. J. Whipp. Manchester University Press, Manchester.

Eyzaguirre, C. and Zapata, P. (1984). Perspectives in carotid body research. *Journal of Applied Physiology*, **57**, p. 931.

Petersen, E. S. (1987). The control of breathing pattern. In *The Control of Breathing in Man*, p. 1. Edited by B. J. Whipp. Manchester University Press, Manchester.

Sinclair, J. D. (1987). Respiratory drive in hypoxia: carotid body and other mechanisms compared. *News In Physiological Sciences*, **2**, 57.

Ward, S. A. and Robbins, P. A. (1987). The ventilatory response to hypoxia. In *The Control of Breathing in Man*, p. 29. Manchester University Press, Manchester.

Chapter 9 Nervous control of breathing

Altose, M., Cherniack, N. S. and Fishman, A. P. (1958). Respiratory sensations and dysponoea. *Journal of Applied Physiology*, **58**, p. 1051.

Bradley, G. W. (1977). Control of breathing pattern. In *MTP International Review of Physiology*, Vol 14, p. 185. Edited by J. G. Widdicombe. University Park Press, Baltimore.

Burki, N. K. (1987). Dyspnoea. *Lung*, **165**, p. 269.

Cohen, M. (1979). 1: Neurogenesis of respiratory rhythm in the mammal. *Physiological Reviews*, **59**, p. 1105.

Coleridge, H. M. and Coleridge, J. C. G. (1986). Reflexes evoked from tracheobronchial tree and lungs. In *Handbook of Physiology, Section 3, The Respiratory System*. Vol II Control of breathing, Part I, p. 395. Edited by J. G. Widdicombe and N. S. Cherniack. American Physiological Society, Bethesda.

Guz, A. (1975). Regulation of respiration in man. *Annual Review of Physiology*, **37**, p. 303.

Hornbein, T. (ed.) (1981). *Regulation of Breathing*, Vols 1 and 2. Marcel Dekker, New York.

Leith, D. E., Butler, J. P., Sneddon, S. L. and Brain, J. D. (1986). Cough. In *Handbook of Physiology, Section 3, The Respiratory System*. Vol III Mechanics of breathing, Part I, p. 315. Edited by P. T. Macklem and J. Mead. American Physiological Society, Bethesda.

Whipp, B. J. (ed.) (1987). *The Control of Breathing in Man*. Manchester University Press, Manchester.

Chapter 10 Special respiratory conditions

Adey, W. R. (1974). The physiology of weightlessness. *The Physiologist*, **16**, p. 178.

Blix, A. S. (1987). Diving responses: fact or fiction. *News in Physiological Sciences*, **2**, p. 64.

Bullard, R. W. (1972). Physiological problems of space travel. *Annual Review of Physiology*, **34**, p. 205.

Dawes, G. S. and Henderson-Smart, D. J. (1981). Breathing before and after birth. In *MTP International Review of Physiology*, Vol 23, p. 75. Edited by J. G. Widdicombe. University Park Press, Baltimore.

Dempsey, J. A. (1986). Is the lung built for exercise? *Medical Science of Sports and Exercise*, **18**, p. 143.

Eisner, R. and Gooden, B. (1983). *Diving and Asphyxia*. Cambridge University Press, Cambridge.

Guilleminault, C. (1987). Obstructive sleep apnoea syndrome. A review. *Psychiatric Clinics of North America*, 10, p. 607.

Hanning, C. D. (1989). Obstructive sleep apnoea. *British Journal of Anaesthesia*, **63**, p. 477.

Heath, D. and Williams, D. R. (1977). *Man at High Altitudes*. Churchill Livingstone, Edinburgh.

Hock, R. J. (1970). The physiology of high altitude. *Scientific American*, **222**, p. 52.

Hornbein, T. (ed.) (1981). *Regulation of Breathing*, Vols 1 and 2. Marcel Dekker, New York.

Mortola, J. P. (1987). Dynamics of breathing in newborn mammals. *Physiological Reviews*, **67**, p. 244.

Phillipson, E. A. and Bowes, G. (1986). Control of breathing during sleep. In *Handbook of Physiology, Section 3, The Respiratory System*. Vol II Control of breathing, Part II, p. 649. Edited by N. S. Cherniack and J. G. Widdicombe. American Physiological Society, Bethesda.

Remmers, J. E. (1981). Effects of sleep on breathing. In *MTP International Review of Physiology*, Vol 23, p. 111. Edited by J. G. Widdicombe. University Park Press, Baltimore.

Rigatto, H. (1989). Control of ventilation in the newborn. *Annual Review of Physiology*, **46**, p. 601.

Sloan, A. W. (1979). *Man in Extreme Environments*. Charles C. Thomas, Springfield, IL.

Wagner, P. D. (1987). The lungs during exercise. *News in Physiological Sciences*, **2**, p. 6.

Whipp, B. J. (1987). Control of exercise hyperpnoea. In *The Control of Breathing in Man*, p. 87. Edited by B. J. Whipp. Manchester University Press, Manchester.

Whipp, B. J. and Pardy, R. L. (1986). Breathing during exercise. In *Handbook of Physiology, Part 3, The Respiratory System*. Vol III Mechanics of breathing, Part II, p. 605. Edited by P. T. Macklem and J. Mead. American Physiological Society, Bethesda.

GLOSSARY

Airways resistance   The resistance to flow of gas presented by the airways of the lungs. Analogous to the electrical resistance of a wire to flow of current.

Alveoli   The blind-ended terminal sacs of the airways where the majority of gas exchange takes place and the majority of lung volume resides.

Anaemia   Literally lack of blood, more usually lack of ability of the blood to carry oxygen due to deficiency of haemoglobin.

Aortic body   Peripheral chemoreceptors situated near the aortic arch.

Apneusis   Breathing with maintained inspiratory efforts

Apnoea   Cessation of breathing in the expiratory position.

Augmented breath   A sigh, a deep breath having an inspiratory duration about one and a half times the normal.

Bohr shift   The displacement of the oxyhaemoglobin dissociation curve to the right so as to release more oxygen as a result of increased levels of carbon dioxide.

Breuer-Hering reflex   Prolonged expiratory pause reflexly produced by lung inflation.

Bronchi   Airways between the trachea and the alveoli.

Carbamino   A complex of protein (mainly haemoglobin) and carbon dioxide which carries about 6 per cent of the carbon dioxide transported by the blood.

Carbonic anhydrase   An enzyme found in red blood cells which accelerates equilibrium of the reaction $CO_2 + H_2O = H_2CO_3$.

Carbon monoxide   A poisonous gas used (in very low concentrations) to measure transfer factor of the lungs.

Carotid body   Peripheral chemoreceptors situated near bifurcation of the common carotid artery.

Chemoreceptors   Areas sensitive to O_2, CO_2 and H^+ in arterial blood which control breathing.

Chloride shift   The movement of chloride ions into or out of red blood cells to compensate for the movement of bicarbonate ions and to maintain electrical neutrality.

Compliance   The ease of stretching of the lungs or chest wall. Reciprocal of elastance. Units = litres. kPa^{-1} or litres. cm H_2O^{-1}.

Conductance   The ease with which gas or liquid can be made to flow down a tube. Reciprocal of resistance.

Critical closing volume   Lung volume at which small airways begin to close due to insufficient external support.

Cyanosis   Blue/grey/purple colour of the skin due to the presence of abnormal amounts of deoxygenated haemoglobin.

Dead space   That part of the lung that is ventilated but not perfused (either 'Anatomical' or 'Physiological').

Diffusing capacity   The ability (capacity) of the lungs to allow gas to diffuse from air to blood and vice versa.

DPG (2,3-Diphosphoglycerate)   Found in red cells, shifts oxyhaemoglobin dissociation curve to the right.

Dyspnoea   The sensation of breathlessness or 'air hunger'.

Elasticity   The tendency to return to normal shape when a distorting force is removed.

Equal pressure point   During forced expiration, that point in the airways at which intraluminal pressure equals external lung pressure and where collapse is likely to occur.

Expiratory reserve volume   That part of the functional residual capacity that can be voluntarily exhaled.

Functional residual capacity   That volume of air remaining in the respiratory system at the end of quiet expiration.

Haemoglobin   A complex molecule by which most of the oxygen in the blood is carried.

Haldane effect   Displacement of the CO_2 dissociation curve upwards in de-oxygenated blood, enabling blood to carry more CO_2 from the tissues.

Henderson-Hasselbalch equation   Equation relating blood pH to blood CO_2 and bicarbonate.

Hyperventilation   Ventilation in excess of metabolic needs.

Hypoxia   Inadequate oxygen supply in body or tissues.

Hysteresis   Characteristic 'loop' shaped graph describing the relationship between two variables where the value of one variable at a given value of the second depends on whether the latter is increasing or decreasing.

Laplace's Law   Law relating the pressure in a sphere of liquid to its radius and the surface tension of the liquid.

Myoglobin   Oxygen-binding molecule, similar to haemoglobin but found in skeletal and cardiac muscle.

Peripheral chemoreceptors   Chemoreceptors sensitive to arterial O_2 and CO_2 tensions and $[H^+]$, found in the carotid body and near the aorta.

Pneumotaxic centre   Respiratory area of the pons whose discharge is thought to cut short inspiration.

Poiseuille's Law   Law relating the flow of fluid through a tube to the pressure drop down the tube and hence the resistance it offers to flow.

Respiratory exchange ratio   Ratio of CO_2 output to O_2 input (also called respiratory quotient).

Respiratory centre   Group of related neurones in the brainstem, discharging with a respiratory rhythm.

Reynolds' number Dimensionless number predicting the characteristics at which lamina flow is superseded by turbulent flow.

Spirometer Instrument for measuring and recording lung volumes.

Surfactant (lung) Phospholipid secreted by Type II alveolar cells which reduces the surface tension of the alveoli and increases lung compliance and stability; dipalmitoyl phosphotidylcholine.

Tidal volume (V_{T}) That volume of air passing into or out of the respiratory system in each breath.

Ventilation ($\dot{V}_{E}$) The volume of air leaving the respiratory system in 1 minute.

$\dot{V}_{A}/\dot{Q}$ ratio Ratio of ventilation to blood perfusion of part or the whole of the lung.

Vital capacity The maximum volume of air that can be passed into or out of the respiratory system in one breath.

INDEX